salon services

THE OFFICIAL GUIDE TO THE CITY & GUILDS
CERTIFICATE IN SALON SERVICES

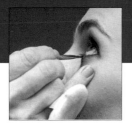 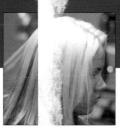 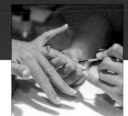

salon services

THE OFFICIAL GUIDE TO THE CITY & GUILDS CERTIFICATE IN SALON SERVICES

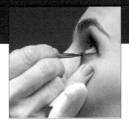 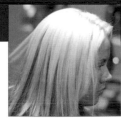 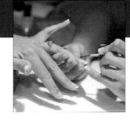

EDITED BY JOHN ARMSTRONG WITH
ANITA CROSLAND, MARTIN GREEN AND
LORRAINE NORDMANN

 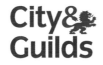 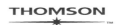

Australia · Canada · Mexico · Singapore · Spain · United Kingdom · United States

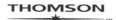

THOMSON

The Official Guide to the City & Guilds Certificate in Salon Services

Edited by John Armstrong with Anita Crosland, Martin Green and Lorraine Nordmann

Publishing Director John Yates	**Commissioning Editor** Melody Dawes	**Development Editor** Elizabeth Catford
Senior Production Editor Alissa Chappell	**Manufacturing Manager** Helen Mason	**Senior Marketing Executive** Natasha Giraudel
Typesetter Meridian Colour Repro Ltd	**Production Controller** Maeve Healy	**Artwork** Oxford Illustrators
Cover Design Harris Cook Turner	**Text Design** Design Deluxe, Bath, UK	**Printer** Rotolito, Milan, Italy

Copyright © 2006
Thomson Learning

The Thomson logo is a registered trademark used herein under licence.

For more information, contact
Thomson Learning
High Holborn House
50-51 Bedford Row
London WC1R 4LR

or visit us on the
World Wide Web at:
http://www.thomsonlearning.co.uk

ISBN-10: 1-84480-456-9
ISBN-13: 978-1-84480-456-6

This edition published 2006 by Thomson Learning.

This publication has been developed by Thomson Learning. It is intended as a method of studying for the Habia qualifications. Thomson Learning has taken all reasonable care in the preparation of this publication but Thomson Learning and the City & Guilds of London Institute accept no liability howsoever in respect of any breach of the rights of any third party howsoever occasioned or damage caused to any third party as a result of the use of this publication.

City & Guilds reserves the right to change the assessment and assignments for this qualification without notice. Course tutors are responsible for confirming that they are using the latest assessment and assignment documents from City & Guilds.

While the publisher has taken all reasonable care in the preparation of this book the publisher makes no representation, express or implied, with regard to the accuracy of the information contained in this book and cannot accept any legal responsibility or liability for any errors or omissions from the book or the consequences thereof.

Products and services that are referred to in this book may be either trademarks and/or registered trademarks of their respective owners. The publisher and author/s make no claim to these trademarks.

British Library Cataloguing-in-Publication Data
A catalogue record for this book is available from the British Library

contents

preface

So you want to be a hairdresser or a beauty therapist?

Choosing our future career is a serious business. We must give it a lot of thought and make sure we have found all the information we need, so we know all about the career we think we want to do. There are lots of questions we need to find answers to, such as: Will I like it? Will I be good at it? Can it provide me with what I need in the future, like a good salary, prospects and opportunities? Perhaps most important, will I be happy in my work if I do this job?

If you are reading this book then it looks as if hairdressing or beauty therapy is something you think you want to do. Taking the City & Guilds 6926 Certificate in Salon Services is a very good way of finding out if hairdressing and beauty therapy is the career area for you and, if so, it will help to set you in the right direction to a fast-track start to your career. Also, if you decide that it is not the route you want to take, a lot of the skills you will get from the programme will be useful and transferable to a wide range of other careers and opportunities.

One thing you will discover very quickly is that hairdressing and beauty therapy are not just about cutting hair and creating styles or doing fancy make-up and giving treatments, but are about developing good personal skills to help you to build relationships with your clients. You will need to be able to provide them with a quality experience and good advice as well as doing the practical work. It takes a lot of time and hard work to learn and develop these skills but they are important to your future.

Hard work starts here, so good luck for a successful career!

John Armstrong

foreword from Habia

Salon Services is an excellent reference tool to support those taking the Salon Services City & Guilds qualification.

The four authors are industry heavyweights, who collectively have an unbeatable combination of all the attributes, experience and styles needed to create this all-encompassing guide.

John Armstrong brings his authority as the Director of Development for 14-16 year olds at Great Yarmouth College, as well as his instrumental role in assisting City & Guilds prepare the Certificate in Salon Services course.

Anita Crosland is an experienced external verifier for the City & Guilds Certificate and is herself an Advanced Practitioner in Beauty Therapy at Bedford College.

Martin Green is an extremely skilled and experienced writer who has worked with Habia for many years. He has a wonderful ability to cater to all learners, from Level 1 to Level 4.

Lorraine Nordmann is also someone who has worked closely with Habia on numerous projects over the years. Lorraine has an abundance of industry knowledge and experience and is an inspirational educator and practitioner.

What impresses me most is the straightforward style that is the key to the overall sense of this book. It gives the reader what they want and need, a real taste of what the hairdressing and beauty therapy industries have to offer them.

I am certain that anyone still considering their options will not be disappointed; rather, they will be inspired and excited about the prospect of joining this fun and rewarding industry.

Alan Goldsbro, Habia CEO

The publisher would like to thank Goldwell Professional Haircare for providing the front cover image for this book.

introduction

ABOUT THIS BOOK

This book is designed to help you study for your City & Guilds Level 1 Certificate in Salon Services.

The chapters in the book are linked to the units that you will take during your course, for example Chapter 4, 'Following health and safety practice', links to unit 004, Following health and safety practice.

The chapters will give you the basic information you need to learn and understand as you work towards your qualification.

Each chapter is broken down into 'bite-size' pieces and each of these contains:

- Clearly explained information that you should read and learn.
- A range of activities that you should complete.
- Boxes containing key facts that are important for you to learn and understand.
- Boxes containing things that you should remember.
- A range of questions for you to answer to help you to see whether or not you have learned what you have read or completed.

At the end of each chapter you will find helpful hints for the assignment for your course.

All the activities that you do can be included with your assignments and portfolio.

ABOUT THE LEVEL 1 CITY & GUILDS CERTIFICATE IN SALON SERVICES

The qualification is made up of nine units. Five of the units are general units and four are practical hairdressing and beauty units.

Units

001 Finding out about customer service
What motivates customers
Different customer needs and expectations
Professional attitudes and behaviour
Working effectively as a member of a team

002 Basic salon reception duties
How to present a positive image of yourself and the salon to the customer
Record and pass on information accurately
Client confidentiality
Different methods of recording appointments
Effectiveness of display areas

003 Personal presentation
How to maintain an alert, natural and confident manner
Present a good personal image
Maintain good personal health and hygiene

004 Following health and safety practice
Develop a positive attitude to health and safety in the salon
Identify potential hazards in the salon
Risk analysis
Fire-fighting equipment, first-aid equipment and accident reporting
Fire and evacuation procedures

005 Introduction to hairdressing services
Preparing the client for hairdressing services
Shampoo and conditioning
Products, tools and equipment
The work area
Drying hair and finishing techniques
Clear, clean and restore the work area
Plait and braid hair
Fashion trends in hair styling

006 Introduction to basic perming and colouring
Preparing the client for perming and colouring
Sectioning and winding techniques
Understanding the perm process
Understanding the client's colour requirements
Selecting product and equipment and preparing the work area
Understanding the colour process
Investigate fashion trends in perming and colouring

007 Applying basic make-up
Preparing the work area
Face shapes and skin analysis
Basic structure and functions of the skin
Reasons for applying make-up
Equipment and products for basic make-up techniques

008 Providing basic manicure
Nail shapes and structure of the nail
Preparing the work area
Equipment and products for manicuring
Manicure procedures
Clear, clean and restore the work area

009 Industry and occupational awareness
Job roles in hairdressing and beauty therapy
Career patterns, training and development
Rights and responsibilities in employment

To achieve the qualification you must fulfil the assessment requirements for each of the units. This will include completing an assignment about the unit, carrying out practical work that your tutor will assess and taking a multiple-choice question paper towards the end of the course. If you successfully complete the assessment requirements of the five generic units, the two hairdressing units and pass the test paper you will achieve the Salon Services Certificate (Hairdressing). If you successfully complete the five generic units, the two beauty units and pass the test you will achieve the Salon Services Certificate (Beauty). Successful completion of all nine units and the test will gain you the Salon Services Certificate (Hairdressing and Beauty).

ABOUT THE CHAPTERS

So that we can see what we have to complete, the first part of each chapter will explain what the unit of the qualification is asking us to do. A further explanation is provided of what we need to find out to complete the assignments and to assist with the practical assessments.

The next part will contain the basic information that we need to know and understand. By learning about what we will be doing in the salon we will understand why we do things in certain ways and what is happening to the hair or the face or body when we do it. This will help us give a better service to the client, be more confident in what we do, work safely and be less likely to make a mistake. We must learn everything we can about the skills we need to develop to be a successful beauty therapist or hairdresser.

Remember what we are learning here is only the beginning of our career. If you decide that this is the career for you then together we can progress to level 2 hairdressing or beauty therapy and then on to level 3 (Chapter 9 will show you how to plan your career). If you do decide that a career in hairdressing or beauty therapy might not be for you, a lot of the skills that you will gain from this book and your course will be transferable and useful in other careers.

ACTIVITY 008–3

Find out the different occasions on which a client might choose to have a manicure treatment and how this might affect the choice of products or colours.

Make sure your tutor has checked your work. Tick when you have completed this activity.

Activity boxes

To help you learn there are a series of activity boxes linked to topics in the chapters. These activities will:

- Make it easier to understand and remember important information.
- Help you prepare for the practical assessments.
- Expand your knowledge.
- Provide evidence for your portfolio.

Not all the activities can be completed from the information in this book. Many of them will require you to search for what you need from other sources. This kind of 'self-directed' learning will broaden your knowledge and understanding of hairdressing and beauty therapy. The activity notes ask you to get your work checked by your tutor, so make sure you do so and then include your work in your portfolio of evidence to support your assignments and practical observations.

REMEMBER

Dispose of all waste products in a lined bin.

Remember boxes

Remember boxes tell us about things that we should remember either because they are fairly important or, in some cases, because they are linked to another topic or chapter.

KEY FACT

Nails grow faster in the summer than winter. Faster in young people than in older.

Key Facts

Important facts are shown in Key Fact boxes. These tell us the important facts that we should make sure we understand and remember. At the end of each chapter is a summary of the Key Facts, just to remind you of the important things.

HINT

Use trade magazines and the internet to help you find out. Look at the job vacancies section.

Hint boxes

The Hint boxes gives you a helping hand to find information, either to help you to complete an activity or to better understand a topic.

Glossary

The Glossary explains some of the important words and titles that are used in the chapter and also provides a handy revision guide. Look out for words written in pink and then check their meaning using the Glossary.

GLOSSARY

Aftercare Information we give to a client at the end of a treatment to advise them on how to improve the condition or prolong the effect of the treatment.

Consultation sheet/record cards Information sheet to record client details and treatment outcomes.

Contra actions A reaction that can happen during or up to 24 hours after a treatment.

Cut out method A procedure used to prevent cross-infection, by using a disposable tool to decant products without having to use your fingers or re-dip into containers.

Effleurage Soft stroking movement.

Formaldehyde An ingredient used in some nail products that can cause severe reactions.

Questions

To help you make sure you have learnt everything you need to there is a short test at the end of the chapter. Part of the test is made up of multiple-choice questions. You should read each question carefully and then look at the four possible answers. Pick the one you think is the right answer and then put a mark against the appropriate letter in the box. The remaining questions are short answer questions. Your tutor will mark these for you.

Helpful hints

To help you complete your assignments for each unit, helpful hints are provided at the end of each chapter to give you some useful suggestions as to how to prepare and then produce your assignment.

City & Guilds reserves the right to change the assessment and assignments for this qualification without notice. Tutors are responsible for checking that they are using the latest assessment and assignment documents from City & Guilds.

Checkerboards

There are checkerboards at the end of each chapter. Use these to help you make sure you have done all the work, that you understand it and that you can describe, list and do everything you to need to be able to do to achieve your goal.

ACTIVITY CHECKLIST

Make sure you have completed all the activities linked to this chapter and that you have put any information you need to keep in your portfolio.

Only tick the box and complete the portfolio reference when your tutor has confirmed the activity is complete.

	Complete	Portfolio Reference
Activity 009–1	☐	
Activity 009–2	☐	
Activity 009–3	☐	
Activity 009–4	☐	

Activity checklist

Each chapter finishes with an Activity Checklist. Use this to make sure you have completed all the activities in the chapter. You should tick each one when you have them checked by your tutor and fill in the portfolio reference when you put the work into your portfolio.

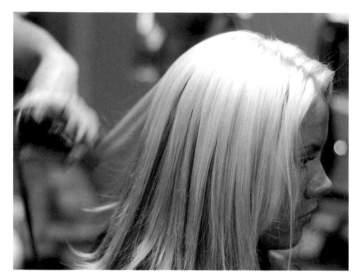 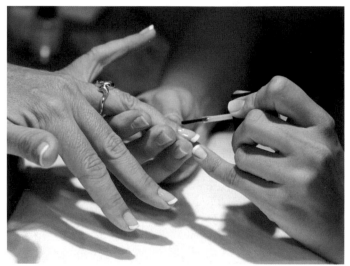

Hairdressing and Beauty Therapy: Hard work but lots of fun!

Well, time to get started! Good luck and don't forget if you want to be successful as a hairdresser or a beauty therapist you will have to work hard but it will be worth it in the end.

chapter 1

UNIT 001 FINDING OUT ABOUT CUSTOMER SERVICE

Introduction

Being very good at cutting and styling hair or carrying out beauty treatments will not guarantee success. Our **clients** want more than just their hair done or their treatment. They want a total experience. So the way we communicate with them, look after them when they are in the salon, provide additional services such as drinks, even the décor of the salon, will be important to ensure client satisfaction and will encourage them to return.

This chapter links 001 Finding out about Customer Service. To help you understand why clients visit a particular salon, what they expect from their visit and what skills over and above your hairdressing and beauty skills you will need to fulfil their expectations.

For the assessment of this unit you will need to show that you:

- **Understand why salons have different 'images'.**
- **Are aware of what things might influence a person to choose a particular salon.**
- **Are aware of a range of things that a client expects from the salon.**
- **Are aware of the need for a personal positive image to be shown to clients and potential clients.**
- **Are aware of the importance of effective communication to the stylist/therapist.**
- **Demonstrate how to communicate in an effective professional manner with clients and others.**
- **Understand the need for client confidentiality and how to maintain it.**

Your assessment for this unit is the completion of an assignment and practical observations.

▶

The assignment will be completed over a period of time and will involve researching information and then putting that information together in a report.

The practical observations will be carried out when you undertake units 005, 006, 007 and 008. (These are the practical units in the programme.) These consist of a series of tasks that you must demonstrate you can carry out effectively and professionally when you do your practical work. Your tutor will observe you carrying out these things and, if you have completed the requirements of the statement, will sign off the task. For the tasks in this unit you will be observed several times before your tutor will finally sign off all tasks. You can gain a pass, credit or distinction in this element. Your tutor will explain what this means during your induction.

WHAT YOU NEED TO KNOW

The assignment will be looking at:

- The images of different salons in your area.
- The reasons why people choose to go to one salon rather than another.
- What impresses people when they visit a salon, what does not impress them, what annoys them and what happens as a result.

For the practical observation part of the assessment you will need to demonstrate, when you carry out your practical work, that you can:

- Speak clearly, politely and appropriately.
- Listen carefully to clients' requests.
- Ask appropriate questions.
- Respond effectively to clients' requests.
- Record details of treatments.
- Relay messages.
- Work as an effective team member.
- Maintain a professional image.

Remember the observation can gain you a pass, credit or distinction.

In addition, you will need to be able to describe the personal skills that a hairdresser or beauty therapist needs to carry out their role.

- The importance of personal positive attitudes.
- How negative attitudes affect others.
- How you can contribute to the work of the team.
- How important teamwork is to the running of the salon.
- The importance of **confidentiality**.

PROVIDING GOOD CUSTOMER SERVICE

Any salon will only stay in business if it has lots of clients who spend money on **services** and treatments. If our salon is going to attract clients and keep those clients then there are a range of things we need to know and do.

We need to find out a lot of information about people's choices and requirements. The questions we need answered are:

- Why do people choose a particular salon? Is it the staff, is it the **décor**, is it the salon furniture, is it the atmosphere, is it because it was recommended by someone else?
- What do they expect from the salon and the hairdresser or beauty therapist? Good cutting, good treatments, good conversation, a happy outlook?
- What would cause them not to visit that salon again? Someone who doesn't pay them any attention, poor cutting, poor treatments, rude staff?

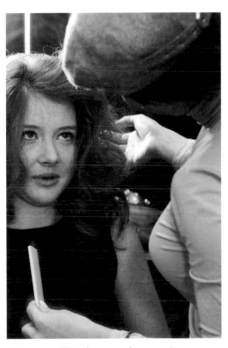
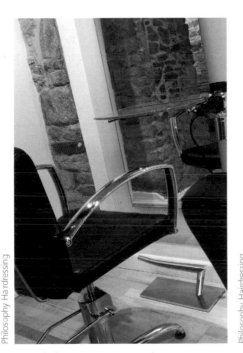
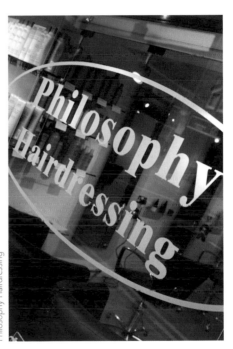

Clients will judge a salon on its appearance and the customer service

The point of finding these things out is that we can make sure we do all the things that the clients like and avoid doing the things they do not like.

Salons are very different even though they generally provide the same services and treatments. Some will be very expensively fitted out, others will not be. Some will be decorated in bright *fashionable* colours others in softer more conservative colours. Some will have *trendy* furniture others more traditional.

This is because the salon wants to create an *image* which it will use to attract clients.

For example if the salon played the latest chart releases, would it attract older or younger clients? Probably younger clients.

When deciding on the image that is required, the salon will want know how people make a choice of which salon to go to. Do they want the cheapest price? Do they want an expensive salon? Do they want bright colours and trendy furniture?

We also need to know what they don't like. Whether it be scruffy looking staff, untidy areas, drab colours or even bright loud colours. If we have some ideas about how people select a salon then we can make sure that our salon meets those needs so the clients will come to us.

The quality of the service, how good their hairdressing treatment or their beauty treatment is, and how we look after them while they are in the salon, will be part of their choosing criteria. Nowadays **value for money** is not far from most clients' minds when they make their choice of salon.

The assignment for this unit looks at three aspects.

The first part of the assignment will help you understand why and how salons are different. It will also help you to consider the personal and vocational skills that you might need to work in a particular salon or type of salon.

The second part of the assignment will help you understand why you must develop *all* the skills you are going to need to be a successful hairdresser or beauty therapist.

The third part should help you understand the importance of people skills. For example, building a relationship with your client and your colleagues, communicating effectively with others, and the quality of your practical work. Another important element you will learn about is the need to look at your own work and make sure it is good enough for the clients and your boss. This is called self-appraisal.

KEY FACT

The ability to communicate properly is a key skill for every hairdresser and therapist.

ACTIVITY 001–2

Write about your own experience of first impressions. Think of somewhere you went and what your first thoughts were about the place (a shop, a club, a restaurant etc.). What influenced your view, was it how it looked, the people, did it look clean etc.? Then in a small group discuss your experience with the others and see what were the common things and what were the individual things. Then as a group write down how, in a salon, could you make sure these were dealt with to give the right image to the client.

Make sure your tutor has checked your work. Tick when you have completed this activity.

REMEMBER

We must know why clients choose a particular salon so we can make sure thjat our salon appeals to clients.

We must know what clients expect so we can provide it.

We must know what would make them not come again so we can avoid doing those things.

FIRST IMPRESSIONS

One of the things you may learn from your assignment is the importance of 'first **impressions**'. We all, when we go somewhere for the first time particularly, will form an opinion of the place very quickly. If a client's opinion is a good one then it will be easier to make them a regular client. If it is a negative impression, then the client is likely to be harder to please when we do their service or treatment.

Think about places you have been to and what impressions you got when you went in.

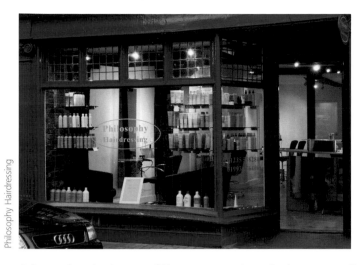

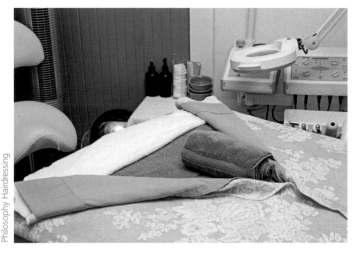

Salons often look very different, even though they generally provide the same services and treatments

When forming an opinion we use all our senses: sight, hearing, smell, touch and taste. We use these to gather information about our surroundings and then analyse that information to form the opinion.

When the clients enter the salon we want to make sure that we present *a positive image* (something that pleases the client) and not *a negative image* (something that does not please the client). We must also remember that presenting a positive image must carry on whenever the client visits the salon. Later in the chapter we will look at the client relationship, how you look after the needs of your client. Another thing we must remember is that even when we are not working on a client we can still affect their opinion of the salon by our actions. If a client can see or hear us then we must present a positive image.

ACTIVITY 001–3

Find out what the words 'positive' and 'negative' mean.

Make sure your tutor has checked your work. Tick when you have completed this activity.

KEY FACT

Always giving the client a positive image when they are in the salon will help to ensure the client is satisfied.

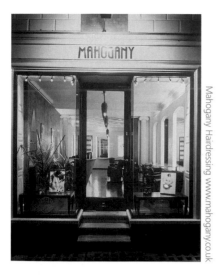

Mahogany Hairdressing www.mahogany.co.uk

NOW TRY THIS

ACTIVITY 001–4

For each of the senses listed, write in the box what would create a positive image and what would create a negative image when a client arrives at the salon.

Senses	Positive image	Negative image
Sight		
Hear		
Taste		
Smell		
Touch		

Make sure your tutor has checked your work. Tick when you have completed this activity.

☐

ACTIVITY 001–5

Answer the question below.

How could you make sure you present a positive image to the client, one that gives a good impression?

Make sure your tutor has checked your work. Tick when you have completed this activity.

☐

KEY FACT !

Everything we do, even when we are not working on a client, must create a positive image.

REMEMBER ✔

Positive images keep clients.
Negative images lose clients.

HINT ★

Think about all the things that the client would see and hear when you are dealing with them.

ACTIVITY 001–6

Find out what the word 'communication' means.

Make sure your tutor has checked your work. Tick when you have completed this activity.

☐

COMMUNICATION

Communicating with our clients and each other is a vitally important part of what we do. If we can't communicate with our clients how are we going to find out what they want? We want people to see us as professional communicators. Professional communication occurs when we deal with our clients and others in a prompt and 'business-like' manner. Polite not rude, friendly not familiar, assertive not aggressive, positive not passive.

Effective communication takes place in the following ways:

- Speech – in what we say to others and the way we say it. This is often called **verbal communication**.
- Listening – by hearing what others say to us.
- Writing – by recording information accurately and clearly.
- Body language – the way we communicate our feelings and attitudes to situations by posture, expression and mannerisms. This is often called **non-verbal communication**.

Think of examples that demonstrate effective communications and poor communications for each of the bullet points listed above.

> **KEY FACT** !
>
> To communicate we use: our voice to speak; our ears to listen; our hands to write; our body to make gestures. The ability to communicate properly is a key skill for every hairdresser and beauty therapist.

Professional communication is being:

Polite

Friendly

Assertive

Positive

Speech

Most of our communication with our clients will be using speech. What we say and how we say it, called the tone of our voice, are very important in giving a positive image to the client about us. Try saying the same phrase to someone using different 'tones' and see if they get the same message. Think about what you are going to say. Saying 'wotcha mate' when the client first arrives will probably bring a negative response, but 'Hello Mrs Smith' will bring a positive response.

It is very easy to forget to be careful about what you say to a client, learn not to forget.

ACTIVITY 001–7

Write down some things that you could say to a client that would create a positive image.

Make sure your tutor has checked your work. Tick when you have completed this activity.

Listening

It is very easy to say 'I always listen to everything anyone says to me'. But in truth we don't, we often only hear part of what people say, or only the parts we want to hear. As a hairdresser or beauty therapist we must listen carefully to everything the client says, particularly about the service or treatment they are having or want. If we don't then we can get things very wrong, with disastrous results. Even normal conversation can be important, if, for example, the client talks about a holiday they are going to have you should remember it and ask how it went when the client visits you again.

Every hairdresser/beauty therapist should have a good memory.

REMEMBER

You must always listen carefully to what your client says to you. You might make serious mistakes if you do not.

Writing

We need to record a lot of information when we are at work. Information about clients' services and treatments, appointments, messages etc. Some salons use computer-based systems for client appointments and records, others have paper-based systems. You must try to gain sufficient IT skills to be able to be trained to use the software the salon has, and you should make sure that your handwriting is clear and easy to read. It could be disastrous if you can't write clearly. For example if you write down the details of a colour process the client had, you will need to give details of the development time of the colour, if your figures are not clear a different colour could result, which will not please the client.

ACTIVITY 001–8

Practise taking messages with a colleague. You should take three messages.

Make sure your tutor has checked your work. Tick when you have completed this activity.

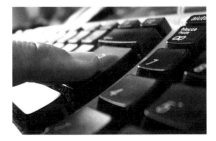

Your salon is likely to use a computerised system for recording information, so basic IT skills will be helpful

Body language

Body language is an important part of communication and is often neglected when we communicate with others. These silent gestures, often referred to as non-verbal communication, convey messages to others.

ACTIVITY 001–9

Try the activity below. Try at least three of your own body language 'messages' and see how many your colleague gets right.

Try this with a colleague
Without saying anything at all try and convey the following messages to your colleague just using body language (hand gestures, body stance, eyes):

- I am very interested.
- I don't believe you.
- It is the truth.

Then try some of your own messages (write them down first).

Make sure your tutor has checked your work. Tick when you have completed this activity.

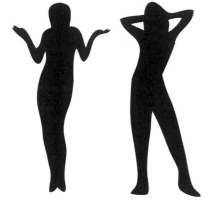

How you hold your body will give others an impression of how you are feeling

A good stylist/beauty therapist can interpret a wide range of unspoken stances and inferences and will always make sure that their body language is giving the right messages to their clients.

Something else we should consider carefully when thinking about communication is answering the telephone and writing or e-mailing people. We can't use all the parts of communication but we still need to present the right image. When you are using the telephone they can only hear your voice the other things that assist communication are not available to them. You should make sure that you speak very clearly and loud enough for the client to hear but not too loud as to deafen them.

Smile when you answer the phone – people will 'hear' the friendliness in your voice.

REMEMBER

You must always be careful about the 'tone' of your voice and what you say on the telephone because the client can't see you.

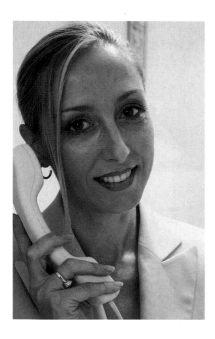

ACTIVITY 001–10

Try the activity below. If you do not have a phone then sit back to back so your partner can't see you.

Try the 'smile' idea out on one of your colleagues to prove it works.

Make sure you repeat the information the client needs so they understand. Remember you will not be able to write it down for them. If you are writing to someone choose your words carefully so they say what you want them to say, are clear, polite and to the point.

Make sure your tutor has checked your work. Tick when you have completed this activity.

Dealing with requests

There will be times when you may not be able to deal with a request or question, and you have to ask someone else for help. This is not a sign of failure or weakness but happens to us all at some time. We can't be experts on everything and sometimes decisions have to be made by someone else, such as the salon owner or manager. Never be afraid to seek help when you need it. It will give the client confidence in you and will make sure they get the best attention and service.

Three other important aspects of good communication are:

- Eye contact. Always keep eye contact with the client when you are communicating with them, it shows you are paying attention to them and not ignoring them.

- Distance. Everyone has their 'comfort zone' (the space around them) and they do not like others to 'invade' that space, they become uncomfortable if it happens. You can find the client's 'comfort zone' limits by watching their facial expression, as you get closer it will start to change. Do not go any closer.

- Not ignoring people. Most people do not like being ignored so acknowledge clients at reception as soon as possible and talk to your client when you are giving the service. People want to see that you are eager to provide a good service, happy in your work, and care about them.

THE CLIENT RELATIONSHIP

When you are with a client give your full attention to them. Use all the methods of communication you need to ensure they get the best service/treatment you can provide at all times.

To do this you will need to show that you want to help and contribute to their satisfaction of the visit. You should convey to them the feeling that you are pleased to see them and really want their business.

The following will help you build a relationship with your client:

- Recognition. Remember people and things about them and then mention those things when they next come to the salon, e.g. if on their last visit they talked about a holiday ask them how it went. Always address your client respectfully, some you will refer to as Mr, Mrs or Miss Smith, younger clients or clients you know well are often addressed by their Christian name. Avoid the use of terms like 'mate', they will generally bring a negative response. As you progress in your career as a hairdresser or beauty therapist you will learn how to 'read' people. This means you will look at their facial expressions, body language and posture to anticipate what sort of mood your client is in and then you can see how to talk to them and what sort of things to say. For example, if they look sad don't say have you had a nice day, they probably haven't.

- Listening. Make sure you make them aware you are paying attention to them and not to others, you should also listen carefully to what they say and the way they say it.

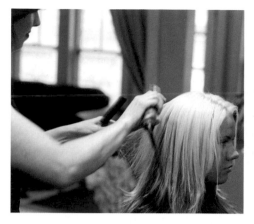
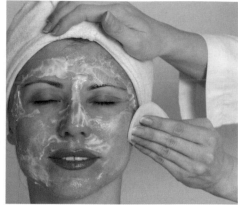

Remember your clients will want a total experience!

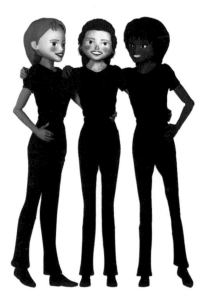

It's not just clients that you will need to build a relationship with!

- Responding. Be positive and confident with your actions. Don't shrug your shoulders, it looks negative, and don't use phrases like 'dunno' (don't know). Be attentive and make sure your client has everything required.

WORKING RELATIONSHIPS

As well as creating good relationships with the clients you also need to create good relationships with your colleagues. Poor relationships with your fellow workers can have a serious impact on the salon. You should always be prepared to help and contribute to the overall team effort. You can do this by:

- Providing support. **Teamwork** is about collectively making an active contribution, by helping each other, even if it is just passing pins and clips or clearing up when others are still working. It helps staff morale and is good for the image projected to the clients.

- Thinking ahead. When you are not busy think ahead as to where there might be things you could do to help others before they have to ask. If a stylist is doing highlights and you think they may not have enough foils (foil pieces used to wrap the hair in) you could either get them for them or ask them if they will need some more and then get them.

- Co-operation. Work together by being aware of everything that is going on in the salon. Be self-motivated, keep yourself busy, don't wait to be asked to do things.

- Maintain working harmony. You can choose your friends but not always the people you work with. You will probably be able to develop good relationships with most of your colleagues but in some cases you will have to work very hard to build a 'working' relationship. Remember that any friction between you and another colleague could create an atmosphere that can be sensed by the clients and affect their satisfaction.

- Respect. All your colleagues have their job to do, respect their skill and knowledge, if you do your job to the best of your ability your colleagues will respect you, and, more importantly, will help you progress.

- Managing your time. Making the best use of your time at work is essential. If you manage your time well things will go smoothly. Poor use of your time, i.e. not pulling your weight, will create a burden for others and rebound on you sooner or later.

Confidentiality

A lot of things that we are told by our clients and many things that we find out about our clients are private. This information must not be told to other people it must be kept **confidential**. Hairdressers and beauty therapists must not gossip with clients. We must not repeat rumours that clients tell us about other people. The way that the salon works and any information, such as the names and details of the clients, are also confidential to the salon. It is likely to be a serious disciplinary matter if this information is passed to someone else. It could cost you your job if you pass on this information.

Respect the client's privacy, don't gossip, don't allow others to do so, and keep all details of the salon's business to yourself.

Developing your career as a hairdresser or beauty therapist will involve looking at what you are good at, what you are not so good at and what you are no good at all at. This is often referred to as your strengths and weaknesses. To become more successful we must maintain and hopefully increase our strengths and deal with our weaknesses by more training and learning. For us it means learning our practical skills and then keeping them up to date. Looking at what the clients want and whether those 'wants' are changing is important. If those 'wants' are changing, we must think about how we must change to meet them.

In the early stages of your career your tutor, supervisor and boss will all measure your performance and work with you to improve. Your individual learning plan is part of this process.

One of things that will help you improve is for you to look at yourself and ask yourself how good are you and what do you need to do to improve your skills. This is not easy because you must be honest with yourself. One question that you should often ask yourself is 'If I had been the client would I have been satisfied with what I have just done'. Another way you can improve is to look at your practical skills and organise things to do to increase your skill level and update your current skills.

The process of thinking about your strengths and weaknesses is called 'self-appraisal'. When your boss, supervisor or tutor does it with you it is called 'appraisal'. You must not look on this as negative or critical, it will be positive and help you develop your career and speed your progress.

The hairdressing and beauty therapy industry relies on people and people can be **unpredictable**. For instance, they don't always do what we expect them to do, they turn up late for their appointment and change their minds about what they want done. Being flexible and able to think quickly and make decisions are essential parts of a hairdresser's or therapist's day. It is at these times that working relationships are really essential.

ACTIVITY 001–13

Write down four things that could be helpful to you if you show others proper respect.

Make sure your tutor has checked your work. Tick when you have completed this activity.

☐

KEY FACT !

Being honest about what you are good at and not so good at is very important if you want to be a good hairdresser or beauty therapist.

ACTIVITY 001-14

When you are doing your practical units think about how you are progressing. Write down what you think you are doing well and get your tutor to comment on it.

Make sure your tutor has checked your work. Tick when you have completed this activity.

☐

KEY FACT !

Being flexible in all aspects of your work is very important to your future success.

Key facts for you to remember from this chapter

- First impressions are an important element in client satisfaction.

- Positive personal attitudes, such as courtesy, patience, good humour, confidence and punctuality, will have a favourable effect on the client.

- Negative personal attitudes, such as rudeness, bad temper, indifference and arrogance, will bring an unfavourable response from the client.

- Hairdressers and beauty therapists must have a flexible approach to their work if they want to be successful.

- Providing the client with the best quality service is key to success.

- The individual's contribution to the work of the team has value.

- Teamwork is vital to success. Working with all people regardless of their ethnic group, age, status and skill level is also important.

- Responding positively to constructive criticism and feedback will help you improve and develop.

GLOSSARY

Client   A customer who pays money for hairdressing or beauty treatments.

Confidential   Information that must not be given to anyone else.

Confidentiality   Not telling private information about someone or something to someone else.

Décor   The style and type of decoration and furniture in the salon.

Impression   How we decide what we think of something from the information we take in from hearing, seeing, touching etc.

Non-verbal communication   Using the body language to transmit our feelings to someone else, e.g. facial expressions (like a smile), hand gestures and the eyes.

Services   The name given to the different things the client will have done. Always used to describe hairdressing tasks, shampoo and blow dry, perm, cut, colour etc.

Teamwork   Working together to get the best results.

Unpredictable   When people or things don't do what we thought they would do, e.g. the client does not turn up for their appointment or turns up late.

Value for money   If the product or service is worth the money paid for it.

Verbal communication   Talking to the client face to face or on the telephone.

Questions to test your knowlege of this unit

Start with these multiple-choice questions. Read the question carefully and then read the four possible answers. When you have decided which of the possible answers is the right one underline either a, b, c, or d in the box under the question.

1 Which of the following does not give a positive image?

   a Politeness

   b Smiling

   c Rudeness

   d Assertiveness

a	b	c	d

2 Which of the following is not part of 'communication'?

   a Speech

   b Resting

   c Listening

   d Writing

a	b	c	d

3 The salon's 'image' will

   a Keep the staff happy

   b Make the salon look nice

   c Look good in adverts

   d Attract the right type of client

a	b	c	d

4 A hairdresser/beauty therapist should always be

   a Very intelligent

   b Flexible

   c Quiet

   d Shy

a	b	c	d

5 Teamwork is important because it

   a Makes the salon more efficient

   b Gives more people a job

   c Means the salon can close on time

   d Gives all the staff a break

a	b	c	d

Questions to test your knowlege of this unit (cont.)

Now try the following short answer questions. These may need a single word to answer or a short sentence or list.

1   Name three things that would give a client a negative image of us and the salon.

Answer   1. _____

2. _____

3. _____

2   Why are first impressions important?

Answer _____

3   Why should you keep eye contact with the client?

Answer _____

4   List three things that should be included in a message taken for someone at the salon.

Answer   1. _____

2. _____

3. _____

5   Give a reason why hairdressers/beauty therapists should have a good memory.

Answer _____

6   What is 'self-appraisal'?

Answer _____

7   Give two reasons why we should ask questions if we do not understand something.

Answer   1. _____

2. _____

Helpful hints for the assignment

Introduction to the assignment

The assignment looks at what you have been learning about in this chapter: the ways that salons present themselves and provide their services.

Like several of the assignments in this qualification, you'll need to look at some salons in your area; if you can, with help from your tutor, visiting them and recording what they are like. So you should be able to collect information for several assignments at the same time.

Your tutor will give you the assignment and guide you on the maximum time you should allow to be sure of completing all of the course assignments.

Picking your salons

Look at all the salons in your area and pick ones that are different: some that are plain and inexpensive, some that are luxurious and expensive and some that are trendy, funky, loud and colourful. Choose which salons you want to research.

Ask the salon if you can visit (get your tutor to assist you). If it is not possible to visit salons then you could find some information in hairdressing and beauty magazines like *Hairdressers' Journal*. You can also do research on the Internet. Don't forget to include a reference to show where the information came from.

Talking about salon images

Think about how you can best describe your salons. Can you take some pictures? What do you need to find out?

Make a list of things you need to find out:

- What is the age range of clients?
- Is the salon furniture ultra modern?
- Are the prices expensive?

Remember to look at the outside of the salon and think about your impression of it.

Making your report

After you have all the information you need, start on the notes. Think about how you can describe the salons you have selected and then make some rough notes. Next think about how you are going to present your report.

Decide whether you want to use a computer or write it by hand, and where you are going to put the pictures. You should start with an introduction; this explains what you are going to do, what you are going to find out. Then your information and pictures. Complete your report with some conclusions, for example, is there a link between the 'image' of the salon and the clients it attracts? Do the funky, trendy salons have mainly young clients?

Why clients choose particular salons: asking about customer service

You will need to ask a range of people why they go to a particular salon. Why did they choose that one in the first place? What sort of things do they like about the salon they go to? What don't they like? Have they ever stopped going to a salon, and if so, why?

It is worth making a list of the things you need to do:

- Make a list of questions to ask
- Find the people
- Analyse the answers.

Asking the questions

Think carefully about your questions, they must ask the right things. You must ask all the people the same questions; if not, you won't be able to analyse the answers.

When you write up your findings, work out how many people said the same thing. That will tell you things such as how important that piece of information is to you as a hairdresser or beauty therapist. For example; if you ask the question 'Do you like your hairdresser to smile?' and all the people say 'Yes', then that is an important thing to remember and to do when you are in the salon.

When you have asked the questions, analyse your answers and then, as with your salon survey, make rough notes, decide how you are going to present them and don't forget your introduction and conclusion.

To finish your assignment

When you have most of your information complete, think about the folder into which you will put it. Think about the design of the front cover. Another useful thing to do is to get someone to read what you have done to see if it makes sense and provides the information asked for.

Remember you must make a list of where you got your information from. If it is from a book then give the name of the book, the author, the publisher and ISBN number (you will find this information in the front of the book).

If it comes from a website then give the website's address (e.g. www.whatever.com). If it is from a salon, then give the name and the owner's name. You don't need to list the names of all the people you asked questions to.

CHECKERBOARD

After you have completed the chapter on Finding out about Customer Service rate yourself on the checkerboard.
(You must be honest with yourself, don't put a tick in the box if you haven't done the work or don't feel that you have learned what you need to know.)

I understand why salons have different 'images' ☐	I am aware of things that clients expect from the salon ☐	I am aware of things that would cause a client to stop coming to the salon ☐	I understand what 'first impressions' are, and how I can make sure I give the right impression to the clients ☐
I know how important a 'positive image' is ☐	I know what professional communication is ☐	I know why teamwork is important in the salon ☐	I know how important body language is in communication ☐
I am aware of the need to keep eye contact with my client ☐	I know the importance of developing good working relationships with my colleagues ☐	I understand why I should show my colleagues respect ☐	I know what 'self-appraisal' is ☐
I know what is meant by strengths and weaknesses ☐			CHECKER BOARD ✓

ACTIVITY CHECKLIST

Make sure you have completed all the activities linked to this chapter and that you have put any information you need to keep in your portfolio.

Only tick the box and complete the portfolio reference when your tutor has confirmed the activity is complete.

	Complete	Portfolio Reference
Activity 001–1 (p. 3)		
Activity 001–2 (p. 4)		
Activity 001–3 (p. 5)		
Activity 001–4 (p. 6)		
Activity 001–5 (p. 6)		
Activity 001–6 (p. 6)		
Activity 001–7 (p. 7)		
Activity 001–8 (p. 7)		
Activity 001–9 (p. 8)		
Activity 001–10 (p. 8)		
Activity 001–11 (p. 9)		
Activity 001–12 (p. 10)		
Activity 001–13 (p. 11)		
Activity 001–14 (p. 11)		

chapter 2

UNIT 002 BASIC SALON RECEPTION DUTIES

Introduction

A hairdressing or beauty salon will only be efficient if it has a well organised and well run reception area. The salon staff may be absolutely brilliant at their work but if the work is not organised efficiently then the salon will not be successful.

This chapter will tell you about how a reception area is run, and how the receptionist or other staff should carry out reception duties.

This chapter links to unit 002 Basic Salon Reception Duties.

For the assessment of this unit you will need to show that you:

- **Understand the need for an efficient reception area and properly trained staff to run it.**

- **Are aware of the need for a personal positive image to be shown to clients and potential clients.**

- **Arc aware of the methods used in salons to record appointments.**

- **Understand the need for client confidentiality and how to maintain it.**

- **Are aware of ways that salons provide information about their services and treatments.**

- **Are aware of the types of products that may be bought at reception and how they can be displayed.**

- **Know what facilities can be provided at reception for clients waiting for services or treatments.**

Your assessment for this unit is the completion of an assignment.

THE RECEPTION AREA

The reception area is usually the first point of contact that clients have with the salon. Their opinion of the salon will be influenced by that first impression. For example, if the area is untidy and dirty looking the client may think that the rest of the salon is also untidy and dirty and that the staff don't care about their work.

First impressions are used by all of us to make judgements about things. If this is so then we must make sure that our reception area and our receptionist give the right first impression to our clients.

What you need to know

As part of the assessment for this unit you will need to:

- Find out about the different systems used in salons to record appointments.
- Find out how salons provide information about their services and treatments to clients and potential clients.
- Find out about the ranges and types of products which can be bought at the reception area and how they can be displayed.
- Be able to describe the facilities that are provided at reception for clients who are waiting for services or treatments.

In addition you will need to be able to describe the personal skills that a receptionist needs to carry out their role.

- The importance of personal presentation when working as a receptionist.
- How a receptionist should communicate with clients.
- How to present a positive personal image to the client.
- How to carry out a financial transaction when the client has had their service or treatment.

Four key statements about the reception area

1 The salon **appointment system** is the efficient way of organising the work for the hair stylists or beauty therapists.

2 *Customer care* is the professional way in which customers of the salon (the clients) are looked after and their needs attended to.

3 *Effective communication* is the process by which information and messages are handled professionally.

4 Confidentiality is the secure way of handling personal information, ensuring only those who are permitted have access to it.

ACTIVITY 002–1

Look at the statements on the left and match them to the statements on the right.
Draw an arrow to link the two boxes that fit.

Make sure your tutor has checked your work. Tick when you have completed this activity.

Retail products should be dusted daily	Because handling information correctly is so important
Hairstyle books and magazines are useful	Because we must convey a professional image and service
Offer clients a drink or magazines	Because they help people describe a new look
Appointment books are essential	Because people don't buy or handle dirty items
Good communication is essential	Because they organise the stylists'/beauty therapists' day
Messages should always be passed on to the right person	Because sometimes they have to wait for a while

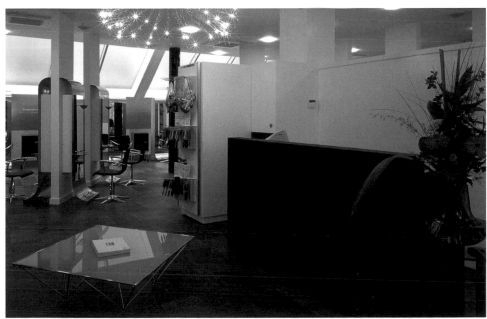

KEY FACT

The appointment system is vital to the salon operation. It must always be accurate, up to date and understood by all the staff.

ACTIVITY 002–2

Find information about one paper-based appointment system and two computerised systems.

Briefly describe how each works and what each does and then say what you think the advantages of each are.

Make sure your tutor has checked your work. Tick when you have completed this activity.

HINT

Use the internet to find information on the computerised systems.

REMEMBER

Doing everything properly is very important when you are on reception.

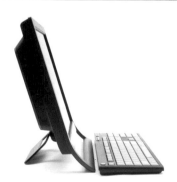

More and more salons are using computer based appointment systems but some still use an appointment book too

THE APPOINTMENT SYSTEM

At the very centre – the 'hub' – of the salon operation is the appointment system. It is the way in which the salon will organise the work that the stylists/beauty therapists do every day. The clients are 'booked' so that they can get the service they require without waiting, and the stylist/beauty therapists can fit in as many clients as they can so they are not waiting for some work to do and not earning any money.

The systems that are used will either be paper based or will be electronic using computer technology. More and more salons are using computer-based appointment systems. Both systems have as their main function details of the work that the staff will do on any day they are working. **Computer-based systems** are able to use that information in lots of different ways to give the salon owner and the staff information to help them assess how well or otherwise the salon is performing.

Find some information about paper-based systems and computerised appointment systems. Describe what each does and how effective you think they are.

Appointments should be made accurately every time, whether the client makes the appointment over the telephone or in person. To do this the receptionist must know all the services offered at the salon. Each salon will have a unique 'menu' of services and prices. These services will take different lengths of times to complete. Different members of staff will have different skills and abilities, they may be able to carry out all the services offered and they may take different lengths of time to carry out the services. The receptionist must know all this information to be able to deal correctly and efficiently with a client.

Making the appointment is not that difficult but it must be done carefully and accurately because the information contained in the '**booking**' will tell the stylist/beauty therapist what they will need to prepare before the client arrives.

The information the receptionist needs to make the appointment is:

- Date and time
- Service/s required
- Stylist/beauty therapist required
- The client's name
- Client contact details

When the information is entered into the system the receptionist will always double check that it is right and meets the client's requirements.

ACTIVITY 002–3

Looking at the list of information we need to make an appointment, think about, and then write down, how you will get what you need to make an appointment.

Make sure your tutor has checked your work. Tick when you have completed this activity.

ACTIVITY 002–4

Do the activity below. Find out the list of services that are offered in the salon and find out the other information. Fill in the chart.

Find out all the services that a salon offers, how long each takes to complete and the cost of each of the services. Remember to find out if there are additional times required for other parts of the service. For example, if the client wants a colour they will also want either a blow dry or another **finishing service** afterwards. There may be a time gap between these parts of the service, make sure you find this out. There may also be other services that link with some you provide.

Service	Time required	Gap required	Cost of service	Other services

Make sure your tutor has checked your work. Tick when you have completed this activity.

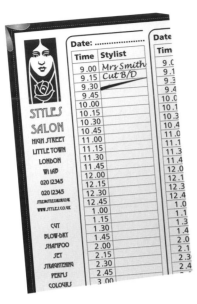

An example from an appointment book

Whether the system is paper based or electronic the process is very similar. This is an example of a page from an appointment book.

ACTIVITY 002–5

Do the activity below. Read the information in the first part and then fill in your appointment sheet with all the clients in the list.

Make sure your tutor has checked your work. Tick when you have completed this activity.

Your salon has three stylists:

- Jane works part time from 1.00pm to 5.30pm.
- Samantha works full time from 9.00am to 5.30pm and has an hour for lunch.
- Tina is a colourist and works part time from 9.00am to 12 noon.

For this exercise use the following service times:

Cut and blow dry	45 minutes
Blow dry	30 minutes
Wet cut only	30 minutes
Dry trim only	15 minutes
Highlights – T section	30 mins plus 30 mins development time
Highlights full head	45 mins plus 30 mins development time
Retouch colour	30 mins plus 30 mins development time

Now read the following information and book the clients onto the appointment sheet.

1 Mrs Cooper, a regular client, has a standing appointment with Samantha for a blow dry at 10am.

2 Mrs Cooper's daughter would like full head highlights at the same time as her mother, with a cut and blow dry with Samantha to finish.

3 Mrs Ford wants the earliest appointment available with Jane for a cut and blow dry and would like to bring her two children for dry trims with whoever is available at the same time.

4 Miss Jones would like a mid-morning cut and blow dry appointment with Samantha.

5 A Miss Collins rings to ask if there is an appointment available to retouch her colour and then a cut and blow dry with Samantha after 10.30am.

6 Mark out time for Samantha's lunch.

7 Two people, Miss Green and Miss Dorkin, call in and ask if there are any appointments available for cut and blow drys as near to 2.00pm as possible, they don't mind who they have but want to have it done at the same time.

8 Someone rings at 1.00pm and asks for their children, Paula and Cherry Tombs, to have a wet cut and a dry trim respectively, before 3.00pm. The person wants to know when they can be fitted in.

Date: _____

Time	Stylist	Stylist	Stylist
9.00			
9.15			
9.30			
9.45			
10.00			
10.15			
10.30			
10.45			
11.00			
11.15			
11.30			
11.45			
12.00			
12.15			
12.30			
12.45			
1.00			
1.15			
1.30			
1.45			
2.00			
2.15			
2.30			
2.45			
3.00			
3.15			
3.30			
3.45			
4.00			
4.15			
4.30			
4.45			
5.00			
5.15			
5.30			

KEY FACT

The quality of service from the receptionist will give the right impression to the client and put them in the right frame of mind for the rest of their visit.

HINT ★

Read the pages on first impressions in Chapter 1, Unit 001 Finding out about Customer Service to refresh your memory.

QUALITY OF SERVICE AND FIRST IMPRESSION

Making sure the client gets the quality of service they will be happy with is very important, especially on reception. The client's first impression of the salon will be gained at reception, if that impression is not a good one the client is likely to find fault in the rest of the service provided even if it is very good.

In Unit 001, Finding out about Customer Service we looked at the importance of first impressions and positive image. When the clients enter the salon they will be taking in information to form that first impression. Think about the things they will be looking at, listening to etc.

ACTIVITY 002–6

Look at the example below and then add your own list of the client's actions when they arrive at the salon. Then say how we could create a positive image and how it could be a negative image.

Make a list of the things that will influence the client's impression of the salon when they enter. Then write down how we could make that a positive image and what would make it a negative image.

Client action	Looking at the reception desk
Positive image	Desk is clean and tidy
Negative image	Desk is untidy, paper everywhere.

Make sure your tutor has checked your work. Tick when you have completed this activity.

☐

HINT ★

Watch what a client does when they enter the salon.

KEY FACT !

Effective professional communication is an essential skill when you are the receptionist.

COMMUNICATION WITH CLIENTS AT RECEPTION

In unit 001 Finding out about Customer Service we also investigated how we should communicate with the clients and others when we are at work. When you are acting as receptionist, effective professional communication skills are very important because of the issue about first impressions.

Let us remind ourselves that when we are communicating effectively and professionally with our clients we are using the following:

- Speech. What we say to others and the way we say it.
- Listening. Hearing what others say to us.
- Writing. Recording information accurately and clearly.
- Body language. Communicating our feelings and attitude to situations by posture, expression and mannerisms.

All of these elements must be performed and used in a really professional manner when you are on reception, to make sure you give the clients the right impression of the salon.

The receptionist should deal with enquiries from clients either in person, 'face to face', or on the telephone in the same way. In both cases we need to respond politely and promptly. Do not leave the client standing at the reception desk while you finish what you are doing and do not let the phone ring for a long time before you answer it.

Give your full attention to the client to make sure you understand exactly what they require. Make sure you speak clearly to make sure you are understood, repeat if necessary. Imagine what would happen if the client arrived on the wrong day or at the wrong time and could not have the service they required.

Good communication is more difficult on the telephone because the client can only hear your voice, the other things that assist communication are not available to them. You should make sure that you speak very clearly and loud enough for the client to hear but not too loud so as to deafen them.

Remember from Chapter 1, if you smile when you answer the phone people will 'hear' the friendliness in your voice. Make sure you repeat the information the client needs so they understand it, remember you will not be able to write it down for them.

When the client arrives for their appointment attend to them promptly, check their appointment and the time and then direct them to a seat. Always make a point of making them feel welcome. Offer a magazine or perhaps a drink and then tell the stylist/beauty therapist that the client has arrived. If they have to wait make sure that they are told and always check that they are comfortable and whether they need anything.

Until you have the knowledge and experience there will be times when you may not be able to deal with a request or question that a client may ask you when they are making an appointment. Ask a colleague for their help. Remember from Chapter 1 this is not a sign of failure or weakness, it will ensure you give the client the right information and make the right appointment, it will give the client confidence in you and they will get the best attention and service.

Don't forget your body language, make sure it matches your verbal communication.

REMEMBER

To communicate well with the client we will use:

Speech
Listening
Writing
Body language

KEY FACT

To create the right impression always give the client your full attention.

REMEMBER ✔

The reception area will give a client their first impression of the salon. Make sure it is a positive one.

KEY FACT

Don't ignore a client when they enter the salon, make them feel welcome.

REMEMBER ✔

If in doubt, ask. It will help prevent mistakes. Your colleagues will respect you for it.

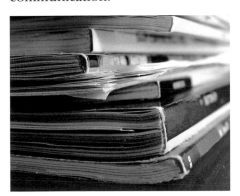
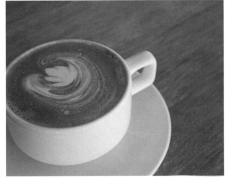

Providing magazines for clients to read while waiting and offering them a drink will make them feel wecome

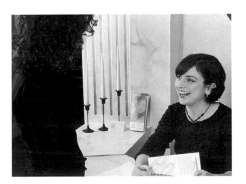

Make sure you give clients the right impression of the salon when working on reception

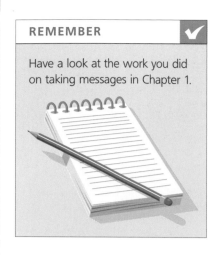
TAKING MESSAGES

The receptionist will at times have to take messages for others, both colleagues and clients. It is essential that these messages are recorded accurately and delivered promptly to the appropriate person. Imagine what would happen if a client telephoned to say that they will be late for their appointment and that message did not get passed on to the stylist/beauty therapist.

When you are taking a message always make sure that you record the time and the date, and make clear who the message is for and who it is from. Then give as much detail relating to the message as you can:

- Who the message is for.
- Who has taken it.
- The date and time received.
- The purpose or the content of the message.

If you have to write the message down quickly while you are taking it, then write it out neatly again afterwards while it is still fresh in your memory.

CONFIDENTIALITY

Remember from unit 001 we must not allow information about clients or anything else to be passed on, or made accessible, to others. When you are on reception speak carefully so as not to let other people overhear easily what you are saying, do not leave papers with confidential details written on them visible to other people. Computer screens can be seen easily by people near to them, make sure that you do nothing that could breach confidentiality.

All salons are likely to have a policy about confidential information. If you disclose that information to others you are likely to be disciplined and possibly sacked as a result.

WHEN THE CLIENT LEAVES

As we have learned the reception area and the receptionist are the first contact the client will have with the salon, they are also the last. When the hairdresser/beauty therapist has finished the services the client requested, they return the client to the reception area for the final part of their visit. The client will pay for the services they have had, we will encourage them to make a further appointment or even appointments and we may introduce them to a range of after-care retail beauty and/or hair products.

PAYING THE BILL

The price we charge the client for the services we provide is the way the boss pays all the bills and wages that allow them to keep the salon open. It is most important to make sure that we calculate the client's bill correctly and then make sure we collect the money and, if necessary, give the right change.

The first part of the process is to make sure the bill is counted up correctly, this may be done using an electronic till or a bill pad and a calculator. If the salon uses a computer-based appointment system then a billing system may be part of it. Make sure you have a list of all the services the client has had. It is important that you do not miss anything out. It will lose the salon profit and make it less successful.

Most salons will accept a variety of payment methods. You should know and understand what they are.

The most common method is cash. There are two things we should remember about cash. Firstly we should make sure the cash is genuine and then we should make sure we give the right change.

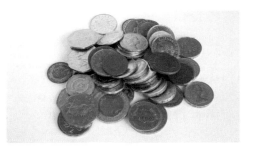
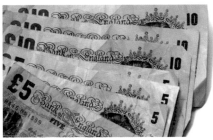

Be careful when taking a client's money and always check to make sure you have given the right change

Other methods of payment are:

Credit or debit cards. As you know no cash is involved in this method but we must make sure we follow the correct procedure so we can claim the money from the bank the client uses.

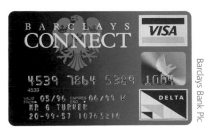

Debit card

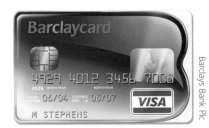

Credit card

Cheques are another form of payment but these are not used as much as they once were. We must make sure the cheque is filled in properly and is validated by a 'cheque guarantee card' so we can claim the money from the client's bank.

HINT ★

Why not impress your client by being able to count up what she has to pay without using a calculator? Learn your maths.

KEY FACT !

Always make sure the client is charged for all they have had. Leaving something off the bill means loss of profit.

ACTIVITY 002-8 ◈

Find out and write down the difference between a credit and a debit card. Find out and write down how a cheque should be filled in correctly.

Make sure your tutor has checked your work. Tick when you have completed this activity.

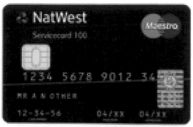

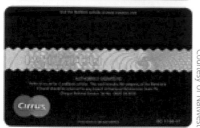

Courtesy of Natwest

Cheque with cheque guarantee card

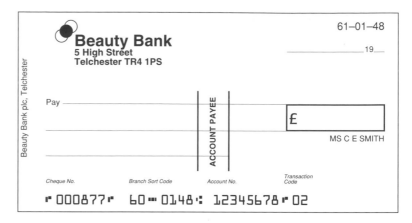

Some salons sell **gift vouchers** that people can give as presents. We get the cash in advance and then give the service when someone comes in with the voucher.

The last method we should be aware of is '**an account**'. This is where a client can have services without paying for them at that time. We provide the services for a period of time, for example a month, and then we send the client a bill for all the services received. This method is often used in hotels where the cost of services is added to the bill for the client's stay.

RETAIL PRODUCTS

Most salons will have a range of after-care products to sell to the clients. The hairdresser or beauty therapist will introduce the client to range of after-care products we sell during the service or treatment. They or the receptionist will try and close a sale when the client is about to leave. The product will be displayed in reception so that the clients can browse when they arrive or leave. A good display of products will encourage the client to buy.

When we have an opportunity we should try and encourage the client to buy products because it increases the money we take, which will in turn increase the salon's profits and our salaries.

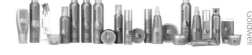

Goldwell

Retail products

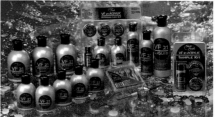

Spangles Nail Art from United Beauty Products

Retail products

ACTIVITY 002-9

Find information about a range of retail products and make a list of what those products are.

Make sure your tutor has checked your work. Tick when you have completed this activity.

☐

HINT

★

Try and find some leaflets about the retail products to include with your list.

KEY FACT

!

No client should leave the salon without a new appointment or without the receptionist trying to sell them a product.

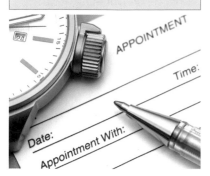

FURTHER APPOINTMENTS

We must try and make sure that every client who leaves the salon has made at least one new appointment. This helps to guarantee our future work and the salon's success. We must also try and sell more services. This can take place at any point during the client's visit but can be more successfully done when the client is making their next appointment.

Key facts for you to remember from this chapter

- The salon will only be successful if the reception systems and the receptionist are efficient.

- Good salons have efficient appointment systems. The staff
have excellent customer service skills. There is good communications between the staff and the clients and between staff and staff.

- Never ignore a client when they enter the salon.

- Make the client comfortable if they have to wait.

- Doing everything properly and accurately on the reception is critical for the salon's success.

- You should know everything about the services offered in the salon when you act as receptionist and engage with the client.

- To create the right impression always give the client your full attention at all times.

- Keep information about clients or things they may have told you confidential. Do not spread gossip.

- At the end of the service make sure the client pays for what they have had and makes another appointment.

GLOSSARY

Appointment system   The way In which clients' appointments for services is kept It tells us what business we are doing on a given day.

Booking   A term used to indicate an appointment. Clients often ask to make a booking rather than to make an appointment.

Computer-based system   A software system for recording appointments and other client details.

Finishing services   Those services that complete the client requirements. For example, after a colour or perm the hair needs to be styled either by blow drying or setting etc. Not usually required in beauty therapy.

Services   The name given to the different things the client will have done. Always used to describe hairdressing tasks, shampoo and blow dry, perm, cut, colour etc.

Treatment   The services carried out in a beauty salon are often called treatments, e.g. manicure, body massage etc.

Questions to test your knowlege of this unit

These are multiple-choice questions. Read the question carefully and then read the four possible answers. When you have decided which of the possible answers is the right one underline either a, b, c, or d in the box under the question.

1 Which of the following would not be part of the information required to make an appointment?

a Date

b Cost

c The client's name

d The client's address

a	b	c	d

2 The appointment system makes sure that the

a salon works efficiently

b staff get a lunch hour

c salon can close on time

d staff can rest between clients

a	b	c	d

3 A scruffy and untidy reception area would

a create a positive image

b create a negative image

c make no difference to the client

d make it easier to work

a	b	c	d

4 Which of the following would not normally be accepted as a method of payment?

a Credit card

b Debit card

c Cheque

d IOU

a	b	c	d

5 When the client leaves the salon we should try to make sure they have

a all their belongings

b left the staff a tip

c made another appointment

d said goodbye

a	b	c	d

Questions to test your knowlege of this unit (cont.)

Now try the following short answer questions. These may need a single word to answer or a short sentence or list.

1 Write down the four key statements about what makes a good reception area.

Answer 1. _____

2. _____

3. _____

4. _____

2 When should we offer the client a drink or magazine?

Answer _____

_____

3 When we make the appointment for a client why would we need some contact details?

Answer _____

_____

4 When we make a telephone appointment why do we need to repeat the information to the client?

Answer _____

_____

5 Write down two things that you need to check when a client pays by cheque.

Answer 1. _____

2. _____

Helpful hints for the assignment

Introduction to the assignment

The assignment looks at what you have been learning about in this chapter: how salons book appointments, provide information about their services and treatments, and present their reception areas.

Like several of the assignments in this qualification, you'll need to look at some salons in your area if you can, with help from your tutor; visiting them and recording what they are like. So you should be able to collect information for several assignments at the same time.

Your tutor will give you the assignment and guide you on the maximum time you should allow to be sure of completing all of the course assignments.

Appointment systems

You will need to find out about some computer-based systems and some paper-based systems for recording appointments.

You can use the Internet to find out about the computer-based ones, but you might need to ask a salon about a paper-based one as they tend to be a basic appointment book that the salon will use as they wish. Decide where you are going to get the information from; you might need to ask people. After you have all the information you need, start on the notes. Think about how you can describe and compare the systems and then make some rough notes.

Planning your report

Just as in the assignment for the first unit, think about how you are going to present your report. Decide whether you want to use a computer or write it by hand, and where you are going to put the pictures. You should start with an introduction. This explains what you are going to do, and what you are going to find out. Then add your information and pictures.

Complete your report with some conclusions, for example, are computer systems best or are they too expensive?

How salons advertise their services

You will need to select some salons – you could look in the local paper for adverts to start you off – and then find out how they advertise. You could ask a range of people how they found out about the salon they go to.

Make a list of the things you need to do:

- Make a list of questions to ask
- Find the salons and people
- Analyse the answers.

Find out what you need to know and then put it together, and as with the appointments report, make rough notes, decide on how you are going to present them and don't forget your introduction and conclusion.

Retail products in the salon

Not all salons sell products to their clients, so you will need to find one that does, to get the information you need. You can also use trade magazines for examples of displays etc. You could use pictures or diagrams to show the products. Then do the same as you did for the other tasks when you write up the information.

Facilities provided for clients at reception when they have to wait

This could link to part of the assignment for the first unit. You may have found out that the reception area is an important part of the whole salon image to attract a particular type of client. You could try to find out if this is true.

Again, follow the same suggestions for completing your report as for the other tasks.

To finish your assignment

When you have most of your information complete, think about the folder into which you will put it. Think about the design of the front cover. Another useful thing to do is to get someone to read what you have done, to see if it makes sense and provides the information asked for.

CHECKERBOARD

After you have completed the chapter on Basic Salon Reception Duties rate yourself on the checkerboard. (You must be honest with yourself, don't put a tick in the box if you haven't done the work or don't feel that you have learned what you need to know.)

I understand the importance of the reception area ☐	I am aware of the ways an appointment is recorded in the salon ☐	I know the four key statements about the reception area ☐	I know that the appointment system is vital to the salon operation ☐
I am aware of the information needed to make an appointment ☐	I know how to make a basic appointment ☐	I understand what the term 'quality of service' means ☐	I know how to make sure the reception area gives a positive image ☐
I know why I should ask for help if I cannot deal with a client's request at reception ☐	I am aware of the need for confidentiality ☐	I know how important it is to calculate the client's bill properly ☐	I am aware of the various ways the client may wish to pay their bill ☐
I am aware that there is an opportunity to sell the client retail products when they leave the salon ☐			**CHECKER BOARD** ✓

ACTIVITY CHECKLIST

Make sure you have completed all the activities linked to this chapter and that you have put any information you need to keep in your portfolio.

Only tick the box and complete the portfolio reference when your tutor has confirmed the activity is complete.

	Complete	Portfolio Reference
Activity 002–1 (p. 21)	☐	
Activity 002–2 (p. 22)	☐	
Activity 002–3 (p. 22)	☐	
Activity 002–4 (p. 23)	☐	
Activity 002–5 (p. 24)	☐	
Activity 002–6 (p. 26)	☐	
Activity 002–7 (p. 28)	☐	
Activity 002–8 (p. 29)	☐	
Activity 002–9 (p. 30)	☐	

chapter 3

UNIT 003 PERSONAL PRESENTATION

Introduction

Our appearance, our dress, hair, nails, and our personal **hygiene** will influence what our clients think about us. We must always try to reflect the desired image of the salon.

In this chapter we will explore how we can always present the right image to our clients and maintain a good standard of personal health and hygiene.

This chapter links to unit 003 Personal Presentation.

For the assessment of this unit you will need to show that you:

- **Understand the need for good personal presentation.**
- **Are aware of the need for a personal positive image to be shown to clients and potential clients.**
- **Are aware of the need for a good standard of personal health and hygiene.**
- **Know the techniques that will ensure a good personal presentation.**
- **Know the factors that encourage personal wellbeing.**
- **Know how to present a good personal appearance.**

Your assessment for this unit is the completion of an assignment and practical observations.

For the practical observations, which will be carried out when you are carrying out your practical hair or beauty work, you will need to demonstrate that you:

- **Carry out your work with confidence.**
- **Always look good, with a professional image.**
- **Always have a good standard of personal hygiene.**

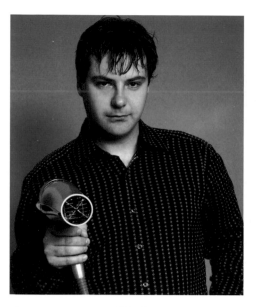
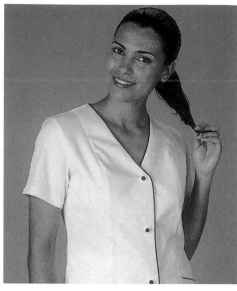

Dream Workwear

Our appearance will influence what clients think of us

HOW WE LOOK TO THE CLIENT

When we are working in the salon our appearance to the client is very important. What we wear will often be decided by our employer. Our clothes should reflect the image of the salon. If our salon is fashionable and trendy, then what we wear should be fashionable and trendy to match.

We must make sure we have a good standard of personal hygiene because we will be working very close to our client, bad breath will offend the client.

We must look after our body and health; it helps us work better and not put clients at risk by transferring illnesses or diseases to them.

What you need to know

For the assignment which is part of the assessment for this unit you will need to:

● Explore different styles of dress or uniform, hair styles, make-up, skin care and nail care, hairdressers and beauty therapists are required to use in the salon.

● Identify the type of salon you would be most comfortable working in.

● Find out whether the 'look' of the staff in the salon affects the way the clients feel.

In addition you will need to be able to describe the various techniques, and reasons for them, to:

● Maintain a good health routine.

● Look after your hands, nails, hair, face and body.

● Present a good appearance.

OUR APPEARANCE

The effort we put into getting ready for work reflects our pride in our work and that we care about what we do. Sometimes we have to wear things that we would not wear if we had a personal choice but professional standards and salon image must come first.

Clothes

What we wear to work will be guided by the image of the salon. But whatever style and fashion we wear it should be practical and serviceable.

Clothes should be easy to clean and iron if necessary and made of suitable fabrics. They should not be tight and restrictive, this would make working harder and more tiring and they may also make you perspire and increase **body odour** (BO).

In the beauty salon we will find that a professional 'uniform' will be the chosen dress code. The services the beauty therapist has to give will require clean hygienic clothing. Beauty therapists may wear a dress, a jumpsuit or a tunic top with co-ordinating trousers, but a clean 'uniform' must be worn every day.

Remember that clothes need washing or dry cleaning regularly and might need to be ironed.

Shoes

Hairdressers and beauty therapists should wear flat or low heeled shoes that enclose the feet (cover the toes). We spend most of our time on our feet so comfortable shoes will help prevent backache.

Hair

As hairdressers our hair is an advertisement of our skill in the salon. If our hair is a mess what confidence does that give our clients? Our hair should always look good and well styled to reflect the salon image.

As beauty therapists our hair should again be well styled but should be tied back off the face and up to the crown if it is long. If hair is of medium length, clip it back so that it does not fall over the face when we are working. The services that we give require bending over the client and if our hair falls towards the client it is unpleasant. Our hair should always be clean, we should wash and condition it when necessary.

Make-up

As a hairdresser if we are going to use make-up it should be complimentary to our hair and dress. If make-up is not used then, like the beauty therapist, we should use the right skin care products to make sure our skin looks as good as possible.

REMEMBER

As a hairdresser your hair is an advertisement for the work of the salon. As a beauty therapist your make-up, or the condition of your skin if you don't wear make-up, is your advertisement.

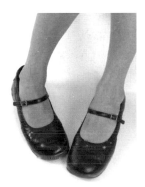

Remember your shoes will need to be comfortable *and* stylish – you are likely to be on your feet a lot

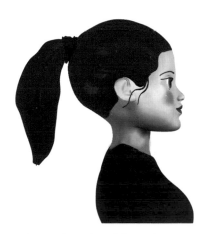

Hair needs to be tidy and presentable

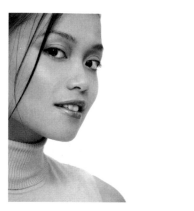

Make-up needs to look attractive

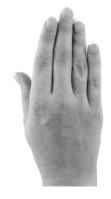

Nails should be smart and tidy and jewellery shoud be avoided

As a beauty therapist our make-up, or if we do not wear make-up the appearance of our skin, is an advertisement of our skills. If make-up is used then an attractive make-up is most suitable. Where it isn't used then use the correct skin care products to improve the condition and the appearance of the skin.

Nails

As for make-up, the appearance of our nails is an important part of our image. The beauty therapist should have short, neatly manicured nails. When working, the nails should be free of nail polish. Polish can be used if our main role is as a manicurist.

The hairdresser should have similar, short, neatly manicured nails. Polish can be worn but must not be chipped or badly applied.

Jewellery

We should not wear too much jewellery while we are working as it can harbour germs, it can be uncomfortable for the client as it can get tangled in the hair or injure the skin.

Hairdressers should wear only a minimum of jewellery. Beauty therapists should not wear any jewellery when they are working on clients (exceptions can be made for a wedding band and small stud earrings).

We must pay attention to all the areas we have just looked at and make sure that we get every area right when we start work in the morning, and check regularly to keep ourselves looking right throughout the day.

PERSONAL HYGIENE

We have looked at our appearance, now we need to look at our personal hygiene. It is no use spending a lot of time making sure our hair and make-up is perfect and then have bad breath because we haven't cleaned our teeth regularly.

Hands and nails

We must make sure our hands are very clean. Not only does it not look nice to the client if they are dirty but it could spread germs to our clients. Our hands are very important to us, they are the way we earn our money so need to be carefully looked after.

If you use chemicals, such as permanent wave lotion, always wear gloves. If you use colour always wear gloves, not only does it protect your skin it will stop your hands from being stained, which does not make your hands look good.

Always wash your hands before work, after using the toilet and after coughing or sneezing, this will reduce the risk of spreading infections.

Use moisturising creams regularly to help replace the moisture lost by constant washing, when you shampoo for example. Sometimes using barrier cream will also help. If the skin on your hands is allowed to become dry it will crack and become very sore, this may prevent you from working until it heals.

Some people may suffer from **dermatitis** from exposure to all the chemicals used in the profession, if your hands continue to be sore and don't heal you should consult your doctor. In some cases a person's sensitivity could mean that they have to give up their job.

Keep your nails clean, especially underneath, and try to keep them neatly manicured and not too long. Check them regularly for any disorders.

Body

The body has sweat glands all over its surface and these are used to help control our body temperature by secreting moisture out on to the surface of the skin when we are hot. This provides a good breeding ground for bacteria which in turn causes body odour (BO). It is essential that we have a shower or bath at least every day and use deodorants, anti perspirants or similar.

Mouth

Unpleasant breath (**halitosis**) can be offensive to others. It can be caused by all sorts of things, from things we have eaten like onions or garlic, which are usually temporary, by smoking, stomach upsets or other problems such as pieces of food that get stuck between the teeth and then decay.

As we will be working very close to our client we will be breathing very close to them and so they will be able to smell any bad breath easily. To prevent bad breath we should brush our teeth regularly, particularly after eating, have regular dental checks and use a mouthwash or breath freshener. Dental type chewing gums work very well but are not appropriate in the salon and should not be used.

Feet

Like our hands our feet are important because we do most of our work standing. We have looked at the sort of shoes we wear and must make sure they fit properly. We should also wash our feet regularly, some people's feet sweat a lot and this can cause foot odour. Make sure minor problems like **veruccas**, corns and **athletes foot** are treated. Some disorders of the feet can make standing painful so we need to get them treated as soon as possible. Toe nails should be cut and filed regularly.

REMEMBER

Looking after your hands is very important. Keep them dry and use hand cream all the time, so your skin does not get dry and cracked.

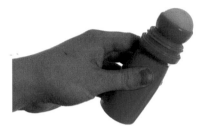

Personal hygiene is as important as making sure your hair, make-up and nails look good

---

REMEMBER

Bad breath can easily offend people. Make sure you don't have bad breath. Don't eat strong foods while working. Don't chew gum.

ACTIVITY 003–2

Keep a diary for a week. Write down all the things that you do during the week that we have said should be in a good health routine, e.g. how many hours sleep did you have every night during that week. Then analyse that information and decide if you have a good personal health routine or not and if not how you could improve it.

Make sure your tutor has checked your work. Tick when you have completed this activity.

☐

REMEMBER

Make sure you don't have smelly feet.

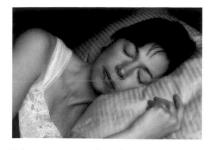

It is recommended that we have 8 hours' sleep a day

PERSONAL WELLBEING

To work successfully as a hairdresser or a beauty therapist you will need energy and stamina. Beauty therapists in particular need lots of energy to carry out massage treatments. Having a good health routine will give us that energy and stamina. The first element of that routine would be a well-balanced diet, one that is healthy and **nutritious**.

We should take regular exercise, perhaps playing sport or dancing. We should also get sufficient sleep and relaxation to help us recover from the stresses of the working day (it is often recommended that we have 8 hours sleep a day). Coping with the stresses of hairdressing and beauty therapy, which at times can be severe, is another thing we must learn to do.

Good posture is a must. As we stand for long periods standing properly will help prevent backache, and in the long term back problems and conditions like **varicose veins**. Always stand with the back straight, your feet apart and your weight evenly distributed on your two legs. Do not stand with all your weight on one of your legs and your pelvis tilted. If you stand like this for long periods you will get backache and possibly more serious problems with your lower back, you will also increase the risk of developing varicose veins.

The care and attention we pay to how we present ourselves for work is very important to our success and progress.

Whatever job we do we should make sure we look the part. Remember different jobs will require us to present ourselves differently. For instance, if you work in an undertakers you could not wear bright, funky, loud clothes.

Being thorough about our personal hygiene will ensure we don't cause offence to anyone else, either to our clients or our colleagues. It can be embarrassing to be told you have a hygiene problem, the best way to avoid this is to make sure you don't have to be told. Having a good diet and enough sleep as part of a good health routine will make sure you can always give your best to your clients, your colleagues and your boss.

Make sure you give enough time to how you look.

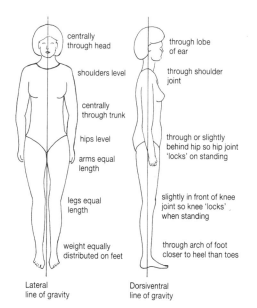

centrally through head

shoulders level

centrally through trunk

hips level

arms equal length

legs equal length

weight equally distributed on feet

Lateral line of gravity

through lobe of ear

through shoulder joint

through or slightly behind hip so hip joint 'locks' on standing

slightly in front of knee joint so knee 'locks' when standing

through arch of foot closer to heel than toes

Dorsiventral line of gravity

Good posture

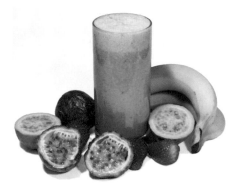

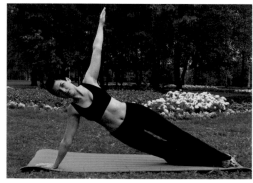

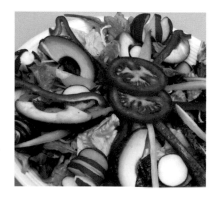

A healthy diet and regular exercise will give you plenty of energy

Key facts for you to remember from this chapter

- Our appearance is a part of the impression we give our clients.

- Our clothes should be appropriate to the salon and the job we do.

- Hair, make-up and nails should create the right impression and reflect the quality of our work.

- Good personal hygiene is important so as not to cause offence.

- Looking after our hands is important to our career.

- A good diet, exercise and enough sleep will give us the stamina and energy we need in our work.

- Good posture will help prevent back problems.

- Check your appearance regularly but not in front of the clients.

- Brush teeth and use a breath freshener if necessary.

- Give enough time to how you look before going to work.

GLOSSARY

Athlete's foot   An infection of the foot caused by a fungus. It is contagious and should be treated as soon as possible.

Body odour (BO)   Unpleasant smell caused by bacteria in sweat.

Dermatitis   A condition that affects the skin. Often caused by being sensitive or allergic to chemicals or other substances.

Halitosis (bad breath)   A condition caused by not brushing the teeth regularly. Caused by decaying food in between the teeth.

Hygiene   The name given to the process of keeping things clean and germ free.

Nutritious   A term used about food items. It means that they are good for you.

Varicose veins   A condition usually seen on the back of the legs. The valves in the veins break down and the veins swell, which can be serious if left untreated.

Verucca   A contagious condition of the foot. They can be painful and should be treated as soon as possible.

Questions to test your knowlege of this unit

These are multiple-choice questions. Read the question carefully and then read the four possible answers. When you have decided which of the possible answers is the right one underline either a, b, c, or d in the box under the question.

1 Which of the following does not give a positive image?

a Politeness

b Smiling

c Rudeness

d Assertiveness

a	b	c	d

2 Which of the following is best for dry skin?

a Soap

b Shampoo

c Moisturiser

d Bodywash

a	b	c	d

3 Clothes worn in the salon should be

a easy to keep clean

b fashionable

c dry clean only

d expensive and chic

a	b	c	d

4 A beauty therapist's nails should be

a short, neatly manicured and with polish

b short, neatly manicured and without polish

c long, neatly manicured and with polish

d long, neatly manicured and without polish

a	b	c	d

5 As a beauty therapist our hair should always be

a worn in a fashionable style

b cut short

c worn back off the face

d worn towards the face

a	b	c	d

Questions to test your knowlege of this unit (cont.)

Now try the following short answer questions. These may need a single word to answer or a short sentence or list.

1 Why should teeth be brushed regularly?

Answer _____

_____

2 What is the best type of shoe to wear in the salon?

Answer _____

_____

3 Write down three things that are part of a good health routine.

Answer 1. _____

2. _____

3. _____

4 What will standing properly prevent?

Answer _____

_____

5 What will influence how you dress at work?

Answer _____

_____

Helpful hints for the assignment

Introduction to the assignment

The assignment looks at what you have been learning about in this chapter: how stylists and beauty therapists dress and present themselves, the kind of salon you would prefer to work in and how the 'look' of the salon affects the way the customers feel.

Like several of the assignments in this qualification, you'll need to look at some salons in your area; if you can, with help from your tutor, visiting them and recording what they are like. So you should be able to collect information for several assignments at the same time.

Your tutor will give you the assignment and guide you on the maximum time you should allow, to be sure of completing all of the course assignments.

How staff dress for work in the salon

Try looking at different salons and the differences in their staff dress and presentation. You could make use of some of the information you collected for the assignment for unit 1 about customer service. Trade magazines could be helpful and you may find some information on the Internet. You could ask a salon if you could take some pictures of the staff.

When you have all the information you need, think about how you are going to present your report. Decide whether you want to use a computer, or write it by hand and where you are going to put the pictures. Start with an introduction and finish with a conclusion or conclusions on what the assignment brief asks for your comments. For instance, did you find that there is a link between how the staff dress and the salon image?

The sort of salon you think you would feel most comfortable working in and why

This should be a brief report, so don't make it too long. When you have decided on the salon you feel would suit you, make some rough notes and make sure you have everything you want to include, then create your report.

Why is staff image and hygiene important to the client?

The final piece of work is about finding out why what we have looked at in this chapter is important to the client. Would they be put off by poor personal hygiene? Is staff appearance something they think about when they are choosing a salon? You will need to ask a range of people for their views. From what they say, make notes on what the task asks you to do. Then do the same as you did in the other tasks when you write up the information.

Did your views change?

Towards the end of your course, you'll be asked if you feel differently about the kind of salon you would be comfortable working in. At that point, you should read what you wrote in answer to this assignment.

If you have changed your mind about the type of salon you would like to work in, then add to your work and write about your new choice. It would be good to give reasons why you have changed your mind. If you haven't changed your mind then you should say that and again say why.

To finish your assignment

When you have most of your information complete, think about the folder into which you will put it. Think about the design of the front cover. Another useful thing to do is to get someone to read what you have done to see if it makes sense and provides the information asked for.

CHECKERBOARD

After you have completed the chapter on Personal Presentation rate yourself on the checkerboard. (You must be honest with yourself, don't put a tick in the box if you haven't done the work or don't feel that you have learned what you need to know.)

I understand why appearance is important at work ☐	I know how to maintain my appearance ☐	I know why my hair and make-up are important to my image ☐	I know why and how to look after my hands and nails ☐
I know why your dress and the type of job you do are linked ☐	I am aware of the importance of personal hygiene ☐	I understand the need to use deodorant to prevent body odour ☐	I know why I should care for my teeth and prevent bad breath ☐
I am aware of the need for a good personal health routine ☐	I know that good posture will help in preventing backache ☐	I am aware of the benefits of a well-balanced diet ☐	**CHECKER BOARD** ✓

ACTIVITY CHECKLIST

Make sure you have completed all the activities linked to this chapter and that you have put any information you need to keep in your portfolio.

Only tick the box and complete the portfolio reference when your tutor has confirmed the activity is complete.

	Complete	**Portfolio Reference**
Activity 003–1 (p. 41)	☐	
Activity 003–2 (p. 43)	☐	

chapter 4

UNIT 004 FOLLOWING HEALTH AND SAFETY PRACTICE

Introduction

The words 'health' and 'safety' are two very important words for anybody who works. You will need to know why these words are important and how they will affect you when you start work. The government has passed a range of laws that an employer (the person or company you work for) must follow to make sure your health is not damaged and that you are not injured when you are at work. Some of the laws apply to you so it is important that you know what you are required to do or not do when you are at work.

This chapter will tell you about health and safety at work. It will cover the **regulations** that you must know about and how you should carry out some of your work.

This chapter links to unit 004 Following Health and Safety Practice.

For the assessment of this unit and for other units you will need to show that you:

- **Understand the purpose of health and safety in the workplace.**

- **Can work safely and professionally, keep your work area safe and tidy, and be aware of others who are around you.**

- **Can recognise possible hazards and their risks.**

- **Are aware of the importance of your own health, hygiene and presentation when you are at work.**

Your assessment for this unit is the completion of an assignment and practical observations when you are doing your practical work.

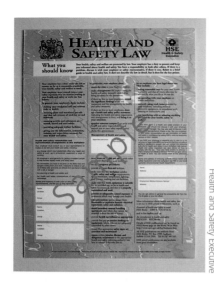

Health and Safety Executive

Health and Safety Law poster

THE HEALTH AND SAFETY AT WORK ACT (1974)

This is the **Act of Parliament** that is the 'umbrella' for all the regulations that concern our health and safety at work. It is sometimes written as 'HASAWA'.

The main aims of the act are to:

- Ensure the health and safety of people while they are at work.
- Protect the health and safety of others from the activities of people at work.

This Act applies to everyone, from those on work experience, people who are employed or self-employed and people who work on contract. It also applies to customers and other people visiting the workplace.

Whenever we are in the workplace and whatever the job we do, our employer must fulfil their responsibilities to us, our colleagues and others on their premises. We in turn must make sure that we fulfil our responsibility to our employer, our colleagues, others on the premises and ourselves.

The following statements are an overview of those responsibilities.

An employer has a legal responsibility to ensure the health, safety and welfare of all people in the workplace.

An employee has a duty not to do anything that may affect their health or safety or the health or safety of others in the workplace.

What you need to know

For the assignment which is part of the assessment for this unit you will need to:

- Show that you are aware of and understand the health and safety requirements of a hairdressing or beauty salon.
- Demonstrate that you can find out who in the workplace is responsible for making sure everything is carried out properly.
- Show that you know what a 'hazard' and a 'risk' are.
- Show what action to take in the event of a fire.
- Show that you can recognise different types of fire fighting equipment and how they should be used.
- Show you understand how chemicals used in hairdressing and beauty treatments should be stored, handled and disposed of etc.

In your practical units you will need to use what you have learned from this unit to:

- Show you can spot hazards and risks and assist in reducing the dangers.
- Show you can carry out your practical work safely and according to the instructions you are given.
- Show you can use products and equipment properly and safely.
- Demonstrate you can follow instructions correctly.

What regulations are part of the Health and safety at Work Act 1974?

There are many sets of regulations that come under HASAWA. The most important ones for hairdressing and beauty salons are these:

1 Workplace Health, Safety and Welfare Regulations (1992)
2 Manual Handling Operations Regulations (1992)
3 Provision and Use of Work Equipment Regulations (1992)
4 Personal Protective Equipment at Work Regulations (1992)
5 Control of Substances Hazardous to Health Regulations (COSHH) (1992)
6 Electricity at Work Regulations (1989)
7 Reporting of Injuries, Diseases and Dangerous Occurrences Regulations (1985)
8 Cosmetic Products (Safety) Regulations (1989)
9 Health and Safety (First Aid) Regulations (1981)

Each of these sets of regulations is about one area of the work we do. You should find out which area they cover and how it affects the way we work by completing the activities in this chapter.

> **REMEMBER** ✔
>
> The key regulations that you should try and remember are:
>
> 3. The Provision and Use of Work Equipment Regulations 1992
>
> 4. Personal Protective Equipment at Work Regulations (1992)
>
> 5. COSHH Regulations (1992)
>
> 6. Electricity at Work Regulations (1989)

HEALTH AND SAFETY POLICY

All hairdressing and beauty salons must comply with all the health and safety regulations. Employers must make sure their staff know how this is carried out.

All employers of more than five employees must have a written health and safety **policy** for that workplace. The policy must be given to all employees and should outline their safety responsibilities and give information such as:

- The storage of chemicals.
- Details of the stock cupboard/dispensary.
- Details and records of checks made by a qualified electrician on the electrical equipment.

> **KEY FACT** !
>
> If you go to work in a salon with more than five staff you must be given a copy of the health and safety policy for the salon.

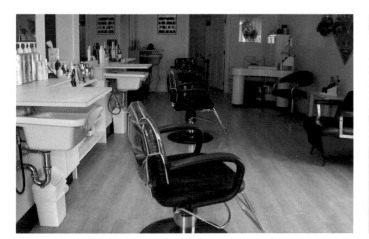
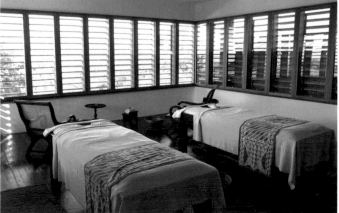

All hairdressing and beauty salons must comply with all the Health and Safety Regulations

- Names and addresses of the key holders for the workplace (people who have a key to the premises).
- Escape routes and procedures.
- Rules on working practices.
- Personal presentation and hygiene.
- Rules on eating and drinking and drug use.

ACTIVITY 004–1

Try and match the regulations on the left with the information in the boxes on the right. Use an arrow to link the boxes.

Provision and Use of Work Equipment Regulations (1992)	Salon chemical products must be stored and kept properly at all times
Personal Protective Equipment at Work Regulations (1992)	Salon electrical equipment must be checked every year
Electricity at Work Regulations (1989)	Moving and handling objects must be done safely and properly
Reporting of Injuries, Diseases and Dangerous Occurrences Regulations (1985)	Information about the use of chemical products
Cosmetic Products (Safety) Regulations (1989)	Box must contain certain items in case of accident occurring at work
Health and Safety (First Aid) Regulations (1981)	An accident occurs in the salon where a client breaks her leg
Control of Substances Hazardous to Health Regulations (1992)	Monitoring of workplace health and hygiene

Make sure your tutor has checked your work. Tick when you have completed this activity.

HINT

To help you use the library, try books such as *The Health and Safety Manual* from HABIA and Croners reference guide to the employer, or try the internet. Using a search engine on the Web type in Health and Safety at Work.

ACTIVITY 004–2

Find out more about the nine sets of regulations listed on p. 63 and what they cover in the salon by making a list as in the example on the below.

In this activity we are going to find out more about each of the sets of regulations. This will help us understand what we have to do in the salon to maintain a safe working environment.

Regulations	What does it affect in the salon.
Personal Protective Equipment at Work Regulations (1992)	The employer must provide adequate protective equipment for the employee to safely carry out their job. Gloves, aprons and towels should be provided for the hairdresser to use and the hairdresser must use them when they carry out their work.

Make sure your tutor has checked your work. Tick when you have completed this activity.

ACTIVITY 004–3

We need to know who in the salon is responsible for health and safety and what we should do in certain circumstances. Finding the answers to the following questions will help us.

Find out the answers to the questions below.

> Question 1. Who has overall responsibility for health and safety in your work environment?
>
> Question 2. What is this person's role in the workplace?
>
> Question 3. If you found something that you felt was not safe in your workplace who would you report it to?
>
> Question 4. What sort of unsafe things do you think you might find? (List as many as you can.)
>
> Question 5. Why are the instructions that come with the products we use important?
>
> Question 6. Who makes sure that the employer maintains a safe working environment and complies with the health and safety law?

Make sure your tutor has checked your work. Tick when you have completed this activity.

ACTIVITY 004–4

Find out what the words 'hazard' and 'risk' mean.

Make sure your tutor has checked your work. Tick when you have completed this activity.

HAZARD AND RISK

A very important area of health and safety for the hairdresser and beauty therapist to know about and understand is *hazard* and *risk*.

Almost anything can be a hazard, but it doesn't have to be a risk. By taking the right action the danger can be reduced. You share a responsibility with your work colleagues for the safety of everyone in the salon including the clients. You need to be able to recognise things that might be dangerous and therefore a hazard and know what you should do if you see one.

Hazards in the salon

Some examples of hazards of the environment are:

- Wet or slippery floors.
- Cluttered passages or corridors.
- Trailing leads or flexes.
- Worn carpets or floor coverings.

Some examples of hazards to do with equipment and materials are:

- Worn or faulty electrical equipment.
- Leaking or damaged containers.
- Badly stored materials.

Some examples of hazards to do with people are:

- Visitors to the salon (clients and others).
- Handling things (stock, furniture etc.).
- Intruders.

ACTIVITY 004–5

Identify the hazards you can see in the pictures and then, in the space provided, answer the two questions about the hazards.

Below you will see a picture of a hairdressing salon and a picture of a beauty salon, study these carefully and identify anything you think is a potential hazard. There are at least ten in each (some hazards may be the same in both pictures).

When you have looked at the pictures answer these two questions about your hazards:

Question 1. Describe the hazards you think are shown in the picture.

Question 2. Do you think the hazard poses a high, medium or low risk to you or others in the salon?

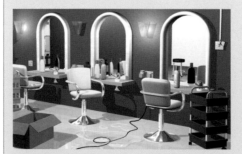

Spot the hazards in this hairdressing salon

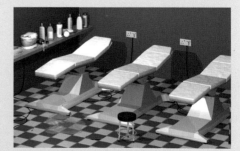

Spot the hazards in this beauty therapy salon

Make sure your tutor has checked your work. Tick when you have completed this activity.

Risk analysis and risk assessment

What you have just done is called risk analysis. This is where you look at the hazard and decide just how likely it is that someone will be injured or damaged by it (whether the risk is high, medium or low).

Risk assessment is where you try to reduce the risk as much as possible by changing how you do things or using other things instead, making it a safer working environment. All salons have to carry out risk assessment on a regular basis to make sure that all risks are reduced as much as possible.

REPORTING HAZARDS

You should always tell the senior member of staff in the salon if you find a hazard. If it is safe for you to deal with the problem then you may be asked to deal with it. As you progress in your job and get more experience then you will take on more responsibility and would be expected to act on your own initiative, but until then always make sure you tell the appropriate person.

Examples of things that you could not deal with are:

- Faulty equipment such as damaged flexes or damaged tongs, dryers or straightening irons etc.
- Loose or damaged fittings such as mirrors, basins, chairs or shelves.
- Obstructions, particularly heavy items that cannot be moved easily.

Some things that you could deal with when told to would be:

- Trailing flexes.
- Cluttered doorways.
- Wet floors.
- Cut hair on the floor.
- Damaged containers.

Find out how you would deal with the hazards in the two lists above. Remember some hazards you can deal with and some you cannot, but you will have to take some action to make sure that no one is injured or affected by the hazard.

As you have found out, spotting hazards is only one aspect of making sure people are not at risk from them. Knowing what the risk of something happening is, is also part of what you need to do.

Look at the hazards in the list below and find out what the risk is if they are not dealt with.

1 Cups, plates and cutlery left out and unwashed over the weekend.
2 Kitchen bleach spilt on to a work surface.
3 Boxes left in reception.
4 Tools not cleaned after use.

KEY FACT

Hazards must be reported. You must not use equipment that is faulty. You should know who to report hazards to.

KEY FACT

Everything we do should be assessed for the risks that may be involved. Before you carry out any services you should check that everything is ok and it is safe to go ahead.

REMEMBER

You should only act within your responsibilities. As you become more experienced and senior, the more responsibility you will have and the more you will need to do.

ACTIVITY 004–6

Find out how you would deal with the hazards listed in the two sets of bullet points on the left.

Include in your answer why you deal with them in this way.

Make sure your tutor has checked your work. Tick when you have completed this activity.

ACTIVITY 004–7

Find out what could happen as a result of the four hazards listed on the left and then add four more from your previous work and do the same.

What is the risk involved from each hazard in your list? Is it high, medium or low?

Make sure your tutor has checked your work. Tick when you have completed this activity.

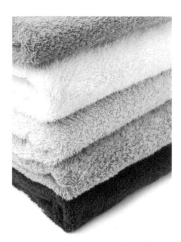
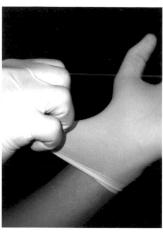
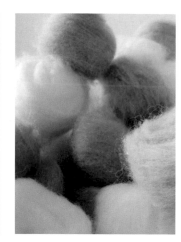
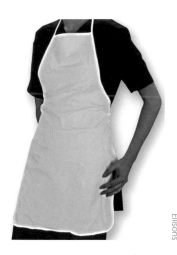

Ellisons

Some examples of Personal Protective Equipment

ACTIVITY 004-8

Find out what each piece of protective equipment in the list on the right is used for and why.

Make sure your tutor has checked your work. Tick when you have completed this activity.

REMEMBER ✔

The Workplace (Health, Safety and Welfare) Regulations are intended to ensure that employees have good conditions in which to work.

ACTIVITY 004-9

Find out what each of the things in the list on the right require the employer to do. See if you can find out what else is covered by the regulations.

Make sure your tutor has checked your work. Tick when you have completed this activity.

KEY FACT !

The employer *must* by law provide the PPE.

The employee *must* use the PPE when they carry out work that requires it.

PERSONAL PROTECTIVE EQUIPMENT (PPE)

Protective Equipment Regulations say that the employer must provide his/her employees with proper protective equipment for use when they are handling chemicals or carrying out dangerous processes. As an employee you need to know when you should wear or use that equipment.

The list below gives some examples of the protective equipment that hairdressers and beauty therapists should use.

- Disposable gloves.
- Waterproof aprons.
- Barrier cream.
- Cotton wool.
- Gowns and towels.

A SAFE WORKING ENVIRONMENT

An employer is required to provide a safe working environment for the employees and a safe environment for the clients. Earlier we looked at the Workplace (Health, Safety and Welfare) Regulations (1992) these regulations cover a range of things that relate to the environment, e.g.:

- The temperature in the workplace.
- The **humidity** and **ventilation** in the workplace.
- Washing facilities.
- Toilet facilities.
- The obstruction of passageways.

Find out more about each of the items in the list.

Another important set of regulations we must be aware of is the Control of Substances Hazardous to Health Regulations, or 'COSHH' as they are often known. You will have found out that these regulations cover safe methods of handling, storing, identification of chemicals and what to do if they are mis-used. Some of the chemicals that are covered by these regulations are:

- Hydrogen peroxide
- Shampoo
- Perm solution
- Hair bleach
- Nail polish
- Skin cleanser
- Moisturiser

ACTIVITY 004–10

1. Find out how the chemicals in this list should be stored.

2. Find out what you should do if the chemicals are misused.

Make sure your tutor has checked your work. Tick when you have completed this activity.

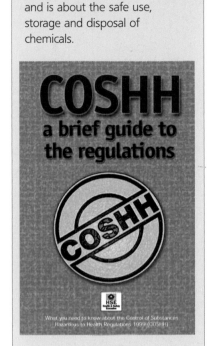

KEY FACT !

COSHH stands for the Control of Substances Hazardous to Health and is about the safe use, storage and disposal of chemicals.

COSHH
a brief guide to
the regulations

What you need to know about the Control of Substances Hazardous to Health Regulations 1999 (COSHH)

COSHH Regulations

HMSO

ELECTRICITY AT WORK REGULATIONS (1989)

These regulations apply to items of electrical equipment. In hairdressing and beauty therapy we use a lot of electrical machines, so these regulations are important to us.

They require our employer to have all the electrical items (including the kettle that we use to make the tea) tested at least every year to make sure they are safe. The test is called a PAT test (portable appliance test) and must be carried out by a qualified person and then marked as passed and detailed records kept. If the item fails the test it must not be used until it is repaired and retested or the item scrapped. We, the employee, must make sure we do not use anything that is not properly labelled or has any faults that are likely to be dangerous to us or others.

THE PROVISION AND USE OF WORK EQUIPMENT (1992)

This ensures that the employer must provide safe equipment for us to use and that the equipment is properly maintained and serviced. The employer must also make sure we are properly trained to use the equipment.

Our responsibility is to make sure that the equipment is safe to use by checking it carefully and not using it if it is not safe. We should also stop anyone else from using it if it is not safe to do so.

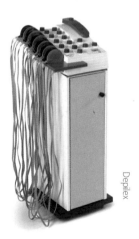

Depilex

An example of electrical equipment you may need to use in the salon

ACTIVITY 004–11

Find an example of an accident report form and write down how it should be filled in. Find out how you would report an accident to the Health and Safety Executive under RIDDOR.

Make sure your tutor has checked your work. Tick when you have completed this activity.

KEY FACT

All accidents must be recorded. *All* serious accidents must be reported to the Health and Safety Executive under RIDDOR.

RIDDOR stands for the Reporting of Injuries, Diseases and Dangerous Occurrences Regulations.

ACCIDENTS

From time to time accidents will occur in the salon. In most cases these will be quite minor, sometimes they will be more serious.

All accidents must be recorded in an accident book that must be kept in the salon. It should contain all the details of the accident, who was involved, how it happened, what action was taken, details of any witnesses etc.

If the accident is really serious then it must be reported to the Health and Safety Executive under the Reporting of Injuries Diseases and Dangerous Occurrences Regulations (RIDDOR).

Accidents can be caused by any of the following:

- Carelessness
- Inappropriate behaviour
- Tiredness
- Misuse of substances (drink or drugs)
- Faulty equipment
- Poorly stored chemicals
- Untidy and dirty work area
- Poor salon layout

FIRST AID

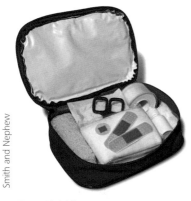

Smith and Nephew

First Aid Kit

The salon must have a first aid box that is properly stocked with all the necessary items needed to deal with minor accidents. The regulations also cover the need to provide qualified first aiders. Find out what materials should be contained in the first aid box.

ACTIVITY 004–12

Make a list of what should be contained in the first aid box.

Make sure your tutor has checked your work. Tick when you have completed this activity.

EMERGENCIES

As well as all the things we have looked at about how we work and making sure that we reduce the risk of harm to ourselves and others, we must also learn about what to do in emergency situations, such as a fire or any other situation where we might need to evacuate the salon.

Fire

The salon or any other workplace must have adequate fire fighting equipment and means of escape. All fire exits have to be clearly marked and exit doors must be able to be opened easily from the inside. They must not be obstructed nor must corridors or passageways that are part of the exit.

The most likely reason for fire occurring in a salon is from an electrical fault, a gas fault (if the salon has a gas supply), or something careless being done by people.

Judith Brown

Some examples are:

- Faulty wiring.
- Badly maintained equipment, both machines used in the salon or in the salon kitchen.
- Gas appliances left unattended.
- Too many appliances plugged into one electrical socket.
- Poorly positioned and unattended portable heaters.
- Smoking.

Your salon will have a set of fire safety procedures. These must always be followed. You should always be aware of what you need to do in the event of a fire wherever you are, at work, staying in a hotel or out for the evening.

At work it is important that you learn the procedure and practise it regularly to ensure that you can get out of the salon quickly when necessary and more importantly, ensure that your clients can also escape safely.

The general rules of evacuation

If a fire breaks out in the salon, the first thing that should be done is to raise the alarm. The person who discovers the fire should immediately tell the person in charge who will then organise the evacuation.

The staff should take responsibility for assisting the clients to evacuate safely. No one should stop to collect anything. The staff and clients should assemble at the assembly point and a senior member of staff should check that everyone is accounted for.

While this is being carried out a designated member of staff will call the fire brigade by dialling 999. If you have to do this then you will need to make sure you have the right information ready to give the operator.

You should never try and fight the fire yourself, unless you have been properly trained to use the equipment and it is safe to do so. If it is safe to do so, all windows and doors should be closed (this will slow down the spread of the fire).

KEY FACT

You must learn the evacuation procedure of your workplace so that you can exit the workplace safely and ensure your clients can also exit safely.

ACTIVITY 004–13

Find out how fire exits should be marked.

Make sure your tutor has checked your work. Tick when you have completed this activity.

ACTIVITY 004–14

Find out the evacuation procedure for your salon (training salon, work experience salon or another work area).

Make sure your tutor has checked your work. Tick when you have completed this activity.

ACTIVITY 004–15

Find out what information you should give the operator if you have to call the fire brigade.

Make sure your tutor has checked your work. Tick when you have completed this activity.

ACTIVITY 004–16

Find out where the fire fighting equipment is situated in your salon. Where are the first aid box and the accident book located?

Make sure your tutor has checked your work. Tick when you have completed this activity.

KEY FACT !

Do not use the wrong type of fire fighting equipment to try to put out a fire.

Do not use fire fighting equipment unless you have been trained to use it.

Fire fighting equipment

Fire fighting equipment must be available and located in specific areas. The equipment should only be used by properly trained people and only when it is safe to do so. It is very important that the right equipment is used. Using the wrong equipment could make the fire worse and endanger the person using it. Different types of fire extinguishers are used to fight different types of fire and they are colour coded according to type. Different types of fire are classified using the letters A, B, C and D according to what materials are involved in the fire.

You should learn how to recognise types of fire extinguisher and be able to classify a fire in order to select the right type of fire fighting equipment. There are four classes of fire:

- **Class A**. Fires that involve solids such as paper, wood or hair.
- **Class B**. Fires that involve flammable liquids such as petrol.
- **Class C**. Fires that involve gases such as propane or butane.
- **Class D**. Fires that involve metals (not normally encountered in the salon).

All fire extinguishers are coloured red but have different coloured labels to show what the contents are. Fire extinguishers will be filled with one of four materials:

- **Water – colour code RED**. These extinguishers are colour coded red and should only be used on Class A fires. *They must not be used on fires involving electrical equipment.*
- **Foam – colour code YELLOW**. These extinguishers are colour coded yellow and are used on Class B fires and small Class A fires. *They must not be used on fires involving electrical equipment.*
- **Carbon dioxide – colour coded BLACK**. These extinguishers are colour coded black and are used on electrical fires and burning liquid.
- **Dry powder – colour coded BLUE**. These extinguishers are colour coded blue and are used on burning liquid and electrical fires.

There is also an extinguisher that contains a substance called BCF Green. These would not normally be used in a salon environment.

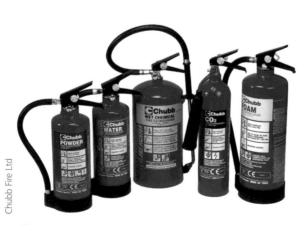

Chubb Fire Ltd

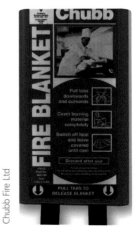

Chubb Fire Ltd

Firefighting equipment

Key facts for you to remember from this chapter

- An employer has a legal responsibility to ensure the health, safety and welfare of all people in the workplace.

- An employee has a duty not to anything that may affect their health and safety or the health and safety of others in the workplace.

- Under the Health and Safety at Work Act there are a range of regulations that must be complied with.

- Personal protective equipment must be used when required. The equipment must be provided by the employer.

- Equipment must be regularly checked and serviced especially electrical equipment.

- COSHH stands for Control of Substances Hazardous to Health and regulates the way we handle, store and deal with any difficulties caused by accidents or misuse of chemicals.

- Employees must be aware of the evacuation procedures to get out of the premises safely.

- Be aware of classes of fire and types of fire extinguishers.

GLOSSARY

Act of Parliament   A set of laws devised by the government of the day and approved by our MPs in the House of Commons.

Humidity   The amount of water vapour in the air, how damp the air is.

Legal   Something that it is lawfully permitted to do or have.

Policy   A course of action to deal with a given situation and usually written down.

Regulations   Similar to laws but usually a set of rules we have to obey.

Ventilation   A flow of fresh air through a room, sometimes natural, such as a window, or sometimes produced by using machines, as in air conditioning.

Questions to test your knowlege of this unit

These are multiple-choice questions. Read the question carefully and then read the four possible answers. When you have decided which of the possible answers is the right one underline either a, b, c, or d in the box under the question.

1 What is the colour code for a carbon dioxide fire extinguisher?

   a Blue

   b Black

   c Red

   d Yellow

a	b	c	d

2 Which of the following should be reported under RIDDOR?

   a A small cut

   b Bruising

   c Broken arm

   d Stomach ache

a	b	c	d

3 Class A fires involve

   a Petrol

   b Butane

   c Wood

   d Metal

a	b	c	d

4 The first thing to do if you discover a fire is

   a Dial 999

   b Evacuate the clients

   c Raise the alarm

   d Close all the doors

a	b	c	d

5 Which of the following is not covered by the Workplace (Health, Safety and Welfare) Regulations?

   a Salon temperature

   b Ventilation

   c Washing facilities

   d Meal breaks

a	b	c	d

Questions to test your knowlege of this unit (cont.)

Now try the following short answer questions. These may need a single word to answer or a short sentence or list.

1 Describe the employee's responsibility under the Health and Safety Act.

Answer _____

_____

2 State two things that should be included in an accident report.

Answer 1. _____

2. _____

3 What information should you give to the operator when dialling 999 to report a fire?

Answer _____

_____

4 Name three things that should be found in a first aid box.

Answer 1. _____

2 _____

3. _____

5 Name two things that we should check on a piece of electrical equipment before we use it.

Answer 1. _____

2. _____

Helpful hints for the assignment

Introduction to the assignment

The assignment looks at what you have been learning about in this chapter; the Health and Safety at Work Act, COSSH regulations and fire and emergency procedures.

Your tutor will give you the assignment and guide you on the maximum time you should allow, to be sure of completing all of the course assignments.

Your responsibilities under the Health and Safety at Work Act.

You will need to find out what your responsibilities are as an employee. You could think about how these responsibilities may change as your career progresses. The second part is about the responsibilities of the employer. These will be more than for the employee; so make sure you cover at least the important ones.

The Internet will be a good place to find out about health and safety. You will need to make sure you get the right information. There are lots of websites you can access and you can print out the information you need.

After you have all the information you need to start making notes think about how you can describe and compare the systems and make some rough notes. Like the assignment for the first unit, think about how you are going to present your report.

Decide whether you want to use a computer or write it by hand, where you are going to put any print outs you want to use. You should start with an introduction explaining what you are going to do, what you are going to find out and then follow with your information. Complete your report with some conclusions, perhaps a brief statement about the employee and employer responsibilities.

Fire, fire equipment and evacuation procedures.

Do a drawing of the floor plan of the salon. The drawing does not have to be to scale but should be a reasonable lookalike. Try to put all the major things that are in the salon on your plan, such as chairs, work stations, basins, windows and doors, etc. Do some rough sketches first and then when you think you have everything you need, then do your final neat drawing. When you mark the things you need to show on your drawing you could use appropriate colours.

Don't forget that there are two other tasks about fire fighting equipment and its use that you need to do. The Internet will be useful to get the information you want, as will the library and advice leaflets, which you may find in a variety of places. When you have all you need, then put it together and don't forget your introduction and conclusion.

A health and safety summary of your salon environment

Use what you have studied in the chapter; such as risk assessment and hazardous situations. You will need to look round the salon carefully and look for things that are hazardous, or could be hazardous if misused. You could use pictures or diagrams to show hazards. Then do the same as you did for the other tasks when you write up the information.

To finish your assignment

When you have most of your information complete, think about the folder into which you will put it. Think about the design of the front cover. Another useful thing to do is to get someone to read what you have done to see if it makes sense, and provides the information asked for.

CHECKERBOARD

After you have completed the chapter on Following Health and Safety Practice rate yourself on the checkerboard. (You must be honest with yourself, don't put a tick in the box if you haven't done the work or don't feel that you have learned what you need to know.)

I know what the Health and Safety at Work Act 1974 is about ☐	I am aware of what the employer's responsibilities are under the Health and Safety Act ☐	I am aware of what my responsibilities are under the Health and Safety Act ☐	I know who is the person responsible in the salon for health and safety ☐
I can recognise hazards and know potential risks in the salon and know how to report them ☐	I am aware of the regulations that apply to me in the workplace ☐	I know why it is important to follow procedures when I am working in the salon ☐	I know why and when I must use personal protective equipment ☐
I am aware of the procedures I must use when using electrical equipment ☐	I am aware of the COSHH regulations ☐	I know what to do in the event of a fire ☐	I know the classes of fire and the colour code of the fire extinguishers ☐

CHECKER BOARD ✓

ACTIVITY CHECKLIST

Make sure you have completed all the activities linked to this chapter and that you have put any information you need to keep in your portfolio.

Only tick the box and complete the portfolio reference when your tutor has confirmed the activity is complete.

	Complete	Portfolio Reference
Activity 004–1 (p. 54)	☐	
Activity 004–2 (p. 55)	☐	
Activity 004–3 (p. 55)	☐	
Activity 004–4 (p. 55)	☐	
Activity 004–5 (p. 56)	☐	
Activity 004–6 (p. 57)	☐	
Activity 004–7 (p. 57)	☐	
Activity 004–8 (p. 58)	☐	
Activity 004–9 (p. 58)	☐	
Activity 004–10 (p. 59)	☐	
Activity 004–11 (p. 60)	☐	
Activity 004–12 (p. 60)	☐	
Activity 004–13 (p. 61)	☐	
Activity 004–14 (p. 61)	☐	
Activity 004–15 (p. 61)	☐	
Activity 004–16 (p. 62)	☐	

chapter 5

UNIT 005 INTRODUCTION TO HAIRDRESSING SERVICES

Introduction

When the client arrives for their appointment, and has been greeted by the receptionist we must escort them from the reception area to the appropriate work station on the salon floor. When the client has been seated they need to be prepared for the services they have booked. In this chapter we will introduce you to the skills and knowledge you will need to prepare the client, assist in the consultation and shampoo their hair. We will also look at conditioning the hair and finishing techniques.

The main assessment requirement for unit 005, Introduction to hairdressing services will be practical observations, where you will carry out the practical tasks we are going to look at in this chapter. There is also an assignment that you will complete. As a result of your practical work and the work we will do in this chapter, which will support your practical work, you will need to show that you are able to:

- **Prepare the work station to receive the client.**
- **Prepare the client for hairdressing services.**
- **Assist in the consultation process.**
- **Select the products, tools and equipment required.**
- **Shampoo and condition the client's hair.**
- **Dry and finish the client's hair using basic techniques.**
- **Clear, clean and restore the work station.**

When we carry out a shampoo, conditioning treatment and finishing service, it is important at all times to follow all the things we learnt in Chapter 4 'Following Health and Safety Practice' and Chapter 1 'Finding out about Customer Service'.

For example you should:

- **Demonstrate how to communicate in an effective professional manner with the clients.**

◀

- **Ask appropriate questions to get any information you need from the client.**

- **Check equipment for faults and your work area for hazards.**

- **Follow procedures when using products.**

- **Record details on the client consultation sheet.**

- **Maintain a professional attitude.**

Remember your practical work will be observed by your tutor and, if you have completed the requirements of the statement, they will sign off the task. For the tasks in this unit you will be observed several times before your tutor will finally sign off on all of the tasks. You can gain a pass, credit or distinction in this element. Your tutor will explain what this means during your induction.

The assignment for this unit will cover a variety of finishing techniques. It involves researching information and then putting that information together in a report.

WHAT YOU NEED TO KNOW

For the assignment which is part of the assessment for this unit, you will need to:

- Find out about different methods of finishing the hair such as blow drying, finger drying etc.
- Find material that shows the effects of these methods.
- Find out what tools and equipment are used in these processes.

For the practical observation part of the assessment you will need to demonstrate, when you carry out your practical work, that you can:

- Get your work area ready for your client.
- Prepare your client for the service they are having.
- Identify the condition of the hair and scalp.
- Get all your equipment and products ready.
- Shampoo the hair using the right procedure.
- Condition the hair, if necessary, using the right procedures.
- Dry the hair by blow drying or other techniques.
- Complete the consultation sheet.
- Finish the service, taking the client to reception.
- Clean the work station.

Remember the observation can gain you a pass, credit or distinction.

This chapter will help you understand what you are learning in your practical work. When we have completed it you should:

- Understand the basic structure of the hair.
- Understand why some conditions may prevent hairdressing services.
- Know the equipment, tools and materials required to prepare the client and work station, to shampoo and condition the hair, to finish the hair and clean and sterilise the equipment and work station.
- Know why and how to shampoo the hair.
- Know why and how to condition the hair.
- Know why and how to finish the hair using blow drying, setting and styling techniques.
- Be able to describe simple braiding and plaiting techniques.

PREPARING THE WORK STATION

When the client is moved from the reception to our work station, where most of the service they will have will take place, it is important that it is clean and tidy. We must make sure that:

- The floor area is clean and free from hair or anything else.
- The chair is clean.
- The mirror is clean with no smudges or dirty patches.
- If there is a shelf it is clean and tidy.
- The trolley is also clean and tidy and everything in its proper place.

Remember our work on impressions in Chapters 1 and 2, make sure the client gets the right impression when they are brought to the salon floor. A clean work area shows a care and pride in your work.

We should not wait until the client is due to arrive to clean and tidy our work station, remember other clients can also see what we do.

KEY FACT

Keeping the salon clean will reduce the risk of transferring infections and diseases. It will also give the right impression to the client.

REMEMBER

If you do not have anything to do then clean and tidy anything that needs it. Teamwork and helping colleagues is important.

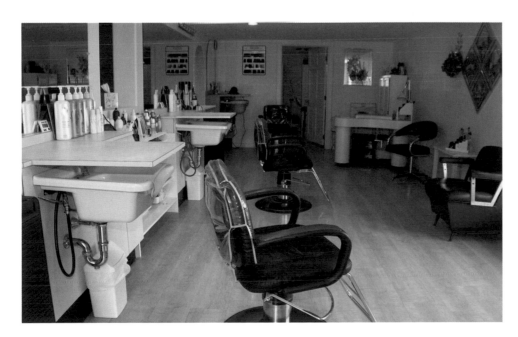

Safe, tidy workstations

ACTIVITY 005–1

Find out more about the methods of sterilisation on the right. Find out how they are used.

Make sure your tutor has checked your work. Tick when you have completed this activity.

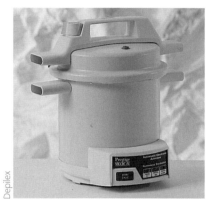

Depilex

An autoclave

KEY FACT

Dirty combs and brushes look awful to the client and increase the risk of spreading infections and diseases.

ACTIVITY 005–2

Find out more about why we have to protect the client's clothes and property when they are in the salon.

Make sure your tutor has checked your work. Tick when you have completed this activity.

The floor should be swept frequently and as soon as possible after cutting hair. Use a mirror cleaner to keep the mirror clean. **Anti-bacterial** sprays can be used to clean work surfaces.

Our tools and equipment must be kept clean and sterilised so as to prevent spreading infections and other conditions from one client to another. This may involve washing them in hot soapy water or using an appropriate method of **sterilisation**.

There are three methods of sterilisation that are used in salons to sterilise tools and equipment.

1 **Autoclaves**. These work like a 'pressure cooker' and the items are heated with a small amount of water under pressure for about 10 minutes. This method will destroy all germs.

2 **Ultraviolet radiation**. This method requires the items to be placed in a cabinet and then exposed to ultraviolet rays from a UV bulb for about 15 minutes. This method is not as efficient as the autoclave.

3 **Chemical sterilisation**. This requires the items to be put into a chemical solution for a short period of time. We must be careful when using this method because the chemical is hazardous to our health. We must use personal protective equipment and remember the COSHH regulations. We often use the name 'Barbicide' to describe this method of sterilisation. This is the brand name of the most widely used chemical steriliser.

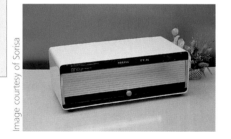

Image courtesy of Sorisa

UV Cabinet

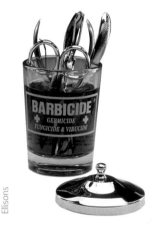

Ellisons

Barbicide

PREPARING THE CLIENT

The first thing we need to do after we have sat the client at our work station is to make sure we protect their clothes from what we are going to do. For this we will need a gown, towels and perhaps tissues or cotton wool.

The gown should be fresh and clean and placed over the client to cover their clothes. A clean freshly washed towel is then placed round their neck and across their shoulders.

Some salons will put a small strip of tissue or cotton wool around the neck as this can stop loose hair from going between the neck and the towel.

It is important that the preparation is thorough because we must protect the client's clothes from damage.

CLIENT CONSULTATION

When we have prepared the client we will need to consult with them about what they want done, so that we can decide how we are going to do it. Until we are experienced enough to do this ourselves one of our colleagues will carry this out with us. In some salons the stylist or cutter will carry out the consultation and then tell us what we have to do for them.

The main purpose of the consultation is for the stylist to assess the quality and condition of the hair and the scalp. The stylist will decide by looking, touching and questioning the client whether:

- The hair is coarse, medium or fine.
- The hair is in good condition or not.
- It is chemically treated with perm or colour.
- Has been damaged by excessive heat drying.

What they will then do is decide whether or not what the client wants can be done. For example, if the client wants a style that requires thick strong hair and they have very fine delicate hair, what they want probably can't be done.

They will also look for any condition or disease that might prevent us from doing what the client wants. The first thing the stylist looks for will be:

- Red inflamed areas on the scalp.
- Scaly rough patches.
- Swellings or lumps and bumps
- Changes to the shape or texture of the hair.
- Anything that does not look like normal skin.

One thing we must all look for is anyone who is infested with head lice. We will look for the egg cases called nits which are cemented to the hair shaft. They look like flakes of dandruff but do not move. The head lice can be

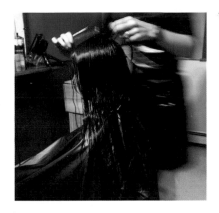

You will need to put a gown on your client to protect her clothes

ACTIVITY 005–3

Find out more about head lice.

Where on the head are they likely to be found?

How should we deal with someone who has them?

How is the condition treated?

Make sure your tutor has checked your work. Tick when you have completed this activity.

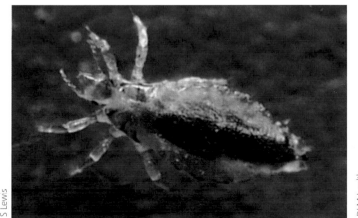

S Lewis

The head louse

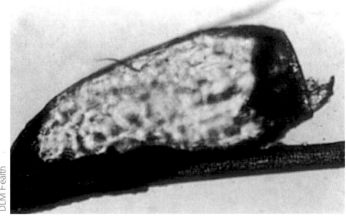

DLM Health

A nit (the egg of a louse)

THE OFFICIAL GUIDE TO THE CITY & GUILDS CERTIFICATE IN SALON SERVICES

REMEMBER

A professional hairdresser is someone who knows everything about the hair and scalp and can advise the client about how to keep it in the best possible condition.

transferred from head to head by sharing combs and other close contact. They can be killed by using a special medicated lotion.

As the condition can be spread, everything that has come into contact with that client must be washed and/or sterilised before it is used on anyone else. That includes us and our hair and clothes just to be safe. We should try and remove the client from the main salon floor as soon as possible so as to avoid embarrassing them and to prevent spreading the condition.

There are many other conditions that you will learn about as you progress through your career. You must learn as much about the hair and scalp as you can. As a professional hairdresser you are probably the only person who can advise the client what to do when they develop or catch a condition or disease. Being a professional hairdresser is not always about just cutting hair.

CHOOSING THE SHAMPOO AND CONDITIONER

In most circumstances the first part of the service will be shampooing and conditioning. So we need to look at the hair and scalp and decide which shampoo and which conditioner we should use, and then the procedure we are going to use.

We should comb the hair to remove any tangles and loose dirt. Comb the hair off the client's face. We should then feel the hair and look at the scalp. Feeling the hair will tell us about its condition, if it feels 'rough' it is likely to be damaged and/or dry, if it feels 'oily' then it is likely to be greasy. To understand this process we need to know the structure of the hair.

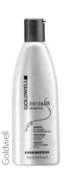 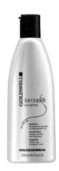 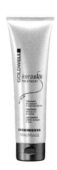 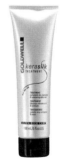 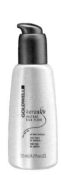

Goldwell

Shampoo and conditioner

ACTIVITY 005–4

Find out some more facts about the three layers of the hair shaft.

Make sure your tutor has checked your work. Tick when you have completed this activity.

THE STRUCTURE OF THE HAIR

A hair is made up of three parts:

1 **The cuticle**. This is the outer layer of the hair. It is made up of see-through flat plates that overlap like the scales on a fish. This layer protects the hair and when the plates lie flat makes the hair shine.
2 **The cortex**. This layer is between the cuticle, which is on the outside of the hair, and the centre of the hair. This area is important to us as hairdressers as this layer gives the hair its shape, it contains most of the colour pigments that make up our hair colour and it gives the hair its strength. This layer can be damaged when we use strong chemicals on our hair.

3 **The medulla**. This layer is at the centre of the hair. It contains some colour pigment and it attracts water.

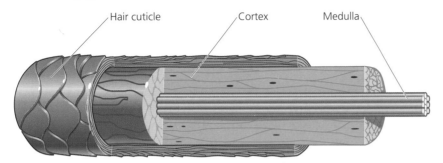

Hair cuticle   Cortex   Medulla

The structure of the hair

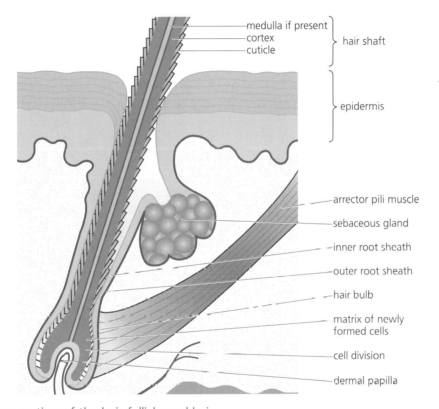

medulla if present
cortex   } hair shaft
cuticle

epidermis

arrector pili muscle

sebaceous gland

inner root sheath

outer root sheath

hair bulb

matrix of newly formed cells

cell division

dermal papilla

A cross section of the hair follicle and hair

The hair grows out of a small 'tube' in the skin called a follicle. The follicle is about 3mm long, at the bottom of the tube is the growing part of the hair. Attached to the side of the hair follicle is a muscle called the arrector pili muscle. This makes your hair stand on end when you are cold or frightened. A gland that produces a substance called sebum, which is the hair's natural oil is also found on the side of the hair follicle. This gland is called the sebaceous gland. If this gland works too hard the hair will become greasy.

ACTIVITY 005–5

Find out more about the follicle, the arrector pili muscle and the sebaceous gland. Try and find out about the skin and what its functions are.

Make sure your tutor has checked your work. Tick when you have completed this activity.

☐

SHAMPOOING

The purpose of shampooing is to clean the hair and scalp of dirt and grease and leave the hair damp and ready for the next part of the service. Water alone will not remove all the dirt particles, we need to use shampoo which contains compounds that are designed to remove them.

We also use massage movements during the shampoo process and these will help the shampoo do its job and it will also improve the blood supply to the scalp, relax the muscles and stimulate the nerves.

As we said earlier, shampooing is often the first part of the hairdressing service. It is therefore very important that it is done properly and well. If we do it well the client will feel that their hair and scalp are clean and they will be relaxed. This will make the rest of the service flow smoothly.

Shampoos come in a variety of forms, gels, oils, creams and pastes. Some are milder and gentler on the hair than others. Some will have different ingredients to do different things to the hair, for example, deep cleansing shampoos for greasy type hair and moisturising shampoos for dry and porous hair. Choosing the right type of shampoo for the hair type and the following service is very important. If we choose the wrong shampoo the hair may become fly away or dull and still feel oily.

Some examples of the types of hair and the shampoo we should use are:

- Hair washed every day needs a mild frequent use shampoo.
- Finer hair needs a gentler or volumising shampoo that doesn't leave it fly away or static.
- Coarse hair needs a shampoo that makes it softer and more pliable.
- Greasy hair should be washed with a medicated or astringent shampoo.
- Dry, porous hair needs a shampoo with added moisturiser.
- Coloured hair needs a shampoo to retain the colour.

When we are ready to start the shampoo process we should take the client to the basin area and ask them to sit. (Some salons have both forward and back wash basins, we would ask the client their preference before we take them to the wash area. If the client has neck or back problems then it may be more comfortable for them to have a forward wash.)

1 Make sure the client is comfortable and that if you are using a back basin that the client's neck is not under any pressure, if it is it could cause injury to their neck.
2 Comb the hair using a large toothed comb to make sure there aren't any tangles.
3 Turn on the water and adjust the temperature. Test the temperature on the back of your hand to make sure it is right for the client.
4 If you are using a backwash place one hand across the hairline at the forehead to stop the water running down the face. Wet the hair from the front hairline to the nape area and the sides, using one hand to prevent water going into the ears or down the front of the neck. If you are using a front wash place one hand across the forehead and push forward as you wet the hair. Use your hands to shield the ears to stop water going into the ears and on to the face.

KEY FACT

Giving the client a good shampoo will relax them and put them in the right frame of mind for the rest of the service.

ACTIVITY 005–6

Make a list of the shampoos that are used in your salon and what type of hair they should be used on.

Make sure your tutor has checked your work. Tick when you have completed this activity.

REMEMBER

Be careful when seating the client at the backwash basin to make sure that the client is comfortable and does not injure their neck.

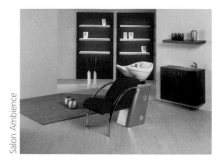

Salon Ambience

An example of a basin area

5 Check the temperature regularly.

6 After the hair is wet, turn off the water, put a small amount of shampoo into the palm of one hand and then lightly rub the hands together and then spread the shampoo over the hair using the flat of the hands.

7 When the shampoo is evenly spread, bend the fingers into a 'claw' shape and use the pads of the fingers to massage the scalp all over for at least a minute. Make sure you don't miss any part of the scalp. Make sure you massage the nape area when you back wash and the forehead area if you front wash.

8 Rinse the hair thoroughly using the same process as you did when you wet the hair at first. Be thorough, rinse *all* the shampoo out of the hair. Also make sure you rinse all the shampoo from your hands especially between the fingers.

9 It is normal to shampoo the hair twice, unless this is not indicated by the condition of the hair and scalp or we are told not to by the stylist. Repeat the process but use less shampoo for the second shampoo. Again turn off the water.

10 We must make sure we rinse the hair thoroughly and remove all traces of the shampoo and gently squeeze out the excess water. Rinse the hands properly.

11 If we do not need to condition the hair then use the towel that is round the neck to form a turban round the head. This will catch any excess water and keep it from running down the client's face or neck. Then sit the client up.

12 Place another towel round the client's shoulders and then gently use the towel round the client's head to remove the excess water from the hair.

13 Take the client back to our work station. Carefully comb the hair using a large toothed comb and starting at the points of the hair at the nape gently comb the hair. Remember the hair will be tangled because of the massage and if you are rough it will hurt the client. Comb the hair off the face, it will be uncomfortable if the client has wet hair on their face.

14 Clean and restore the basin area ready for the next client.

There are three types of massage movements used when we shampoo, they are:

Effleurage – this is a soft stroking movement that we use to spread the shampoo on to the hair or when we do not want to stimulate the scalp.

Rotary – this is the name of the movement with the pads of the fingers held in a claw like fashion. We press the pads quite firmly on to the scalp and then move the hands in small circles all over the scalp.

Friction – this is the same as the rotary movement but carried out with more speed and slightly more pressure.

There is another massage movement called pettrisage which can be used when we are conditioning the hair. Pettrisage is a slow deep kneading movement.

ACTIVITY 005–7

Find out why you need to test the temperature of the water on the back of your hand.

Make sure your tutor has checked your work. Tick when you have completed this activity.

☐

REMEMBER

Only use as much shampoo as you need, to avoid waste. Short hair needs less than long hair.

REMEMBER ✔

When you shampoo make sure you rinse the shampoo off your hands and dry them thoroughly especially between the fingers. Use hand cream regularly to keep the skin from drying out and cracking.

KEY FACT

The massage movements used in shampooing are:

Effleurage – soft stroking movement.

Rotary – a stronger stimulating movement.

Friction – a stronger version of rotary massage.

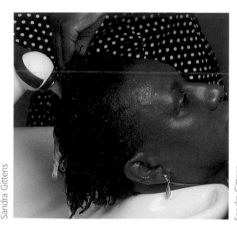
Sandra Gittens

Wetting the hair

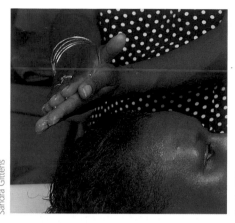
Sandra Gittens

Spreading shampoo over the palms

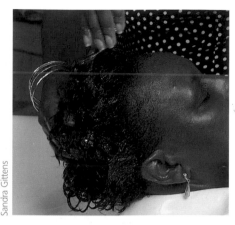
Sandra Gittens

Distributing the shampoo throughout the hair using effleurage movements

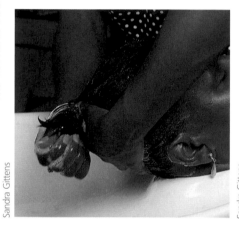
Sandra Gittens

Distributing the shampoo throughout the hair using effleurage movements.

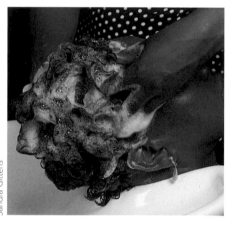
Sandra Gittens

Pushing the fingers under the hair and massaging the scalp

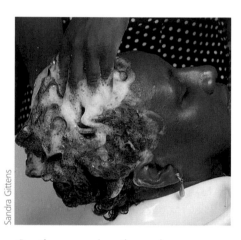
Sandra Gittens

Gently massaging the scalp

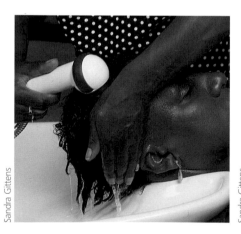
Sandra Gittens

Rinsing the hair

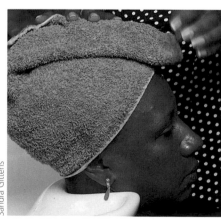
Sandra Gittens

Wrapping a towel round the hair

Thanks to Sandra Gittens, author of *African Caribbean Hairdressing* and Vinetta McIntosh, Lecturer, for the use of images

CONDITIONING THE HAIR

If the hair is dry and/or damaged it will not look its best when we have finished the service. We will need to use a conditioning product which will:

- Allow the hair to be softened and made more flexible.
- Allow the hair cuticle to be smoothed.
- Make the hair easier to comb and detangle.
- Temporarily 'repair' damaged hair.
- Give the hair back its natural chemical balance.

If the hair is dry or just damaged by general wear and tear then a general purpose conditioner can be used. This will smooth the cuticle and soften the hair, which will make the hair shine after the finishing service.

If the hair has been chemically treated or seriously damaged by heat processes then a deep penetrating, more specific conditioner will be used.

If a conditioner is going to be used then it will be applied to the hair after the shampoo.

1 When the hair has been rinsed clear of shampoo, squeeze the excess water from the hair.

2 Put a small amount of conditioner on to the palm of one hand and then rub the hands together and using the effleurage movement spread the conditioner over the hair.

3 If the hair is long, rub the conditioner on to the lengths of the hair first and then to the 'root' area.

4 Massage the conditioner into the hair using either the rotary movement or the pettrissage movement, for at least 2 minutes. The poorer the condition of the hair the longer the massage should be. It can be helpful to comb the hair with a large toothed comb before rinsing the conditioner out of the hair.

5 Rinse the conditioner from the hair as you did with the shampoo.

6 Squeeze the excess water from the hair and then use the towel as you did for the shampoo.

7 Take the client back to your work station and comb the hair carefully and always off the face.

Some specialised conditioners will be used in different ways to this. The stylist will tell us what we need to do if a change is necessary.

ACTIVITY 005–8

Find out two other methods of carrying out a conditioning treatment on the hair.

Make sure your tutor has checked your work. Tick when you have completed this activity.

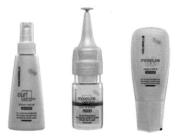

A range of conditioning treatments

Goldwell

FINISHING TECHNIQUES

In this part of the chapter we are going to look at finishing techniques. Basic blow drying techniques, roller setting, plaiting and braiding.

When the other parts of the service have been finished or the client just wants their hair washed and dried then we will use a wide variety of techniques to style the hair to improve its appearance.

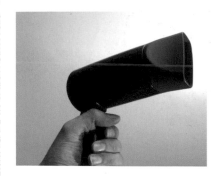

Hand dryer

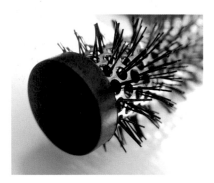

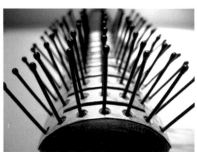

Brushes

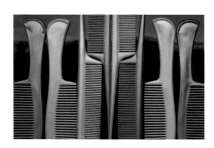

Combs

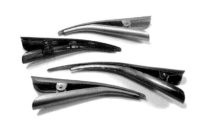

Sectioning clips

Basic blow drying techniques

This is the process of styling wet hair while blow drying it. Using a hand-held dryer we mould the hair using brushes, combs or the fingers, positioning it to fit the style that the hair has been cut to. The tools we can use include:

- The hand-held dryer. These come in a wide variety of models. The dryer should have controls for temperature and speed of air flow. Choose one that is easy to handle and that has the controls in easy reach when you are using it.

- Hand dryer attachments. These will generally be the **nozzle** and the **diffuser**. The nozzle will be used when we want to direct the flow of air in a particular direction or place, we usually use it to blow dry a wave movement or lift into the hair. The diffuser will spread the airflow over a wider area; it is used when we do not want to move the hair too much, it is often used when finger or scrunch drying.

- Brushes. After the dryer the brush is the most important piece of equipment we need. They come in a huge variety of types and shapes. We choose them to our personal taste but the general types will do specific things to the hair. Most of these brushes are firm and with stiff plastic bristles (teeth). Soft brushes are not used for blow drying. A half round plastic brush (often called a 'denman' after the name of the makers) is used for general shaping. Larger for longer hair, smaller for shorter hair. A range of round roller brushes with semi-stiff short bristles are used for a variety of effects, such as curls and volume.

- Combs. These, like brushes come in a wide variety of shapes and sizes. For drying we would normally use a comb that has both widely spaced and narrowly spaced teeth. A large very widely spaced comb is often used after blow drying to achieve a soft look to the hair.

- Sectioning clips. These are large clips that are used to hold the hair in sections out of the way while you blow dry.

We can use these tools to dry the hair in a variety of ways:

- Blow Drying. Drying the hair with the hand-held dryer into a chosen shape or required direction using a brush.

- Blow waving. Shaping the hair into waves using directed air from the drier with a fitted nozzle, using either a comb or brush.

- Scrunch drying. Drying the hair using a hand-held dryer with a diffuser attached and using the fingers to squeeze clumps of hair into a casual rumpled moulded shape.

- Finger drying. This uses the fingers to lift, direct and tease the hair into the shape required. Achieves casual soft flowing styles.

Blow drying

We can start blow drying on any part of the head. On long hair it is best to dry the lower underneath section first. Do not allow wet sections to fall on to the lower previously dried ones. Blow drying works best on coarse hair, fine hair may get overdried and is more difficult to control.

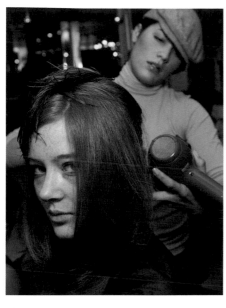

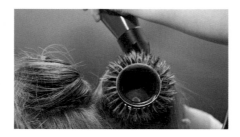

Blow waving

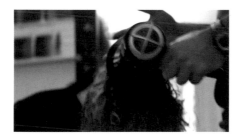

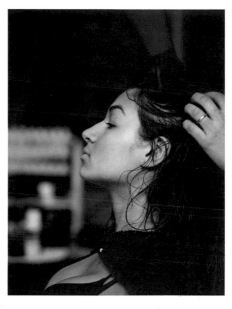

Blow drying

Scrunch drying

Finger drying

Which brush or other tools we use depends on the style effects we want to achieve, as you gain in experience you will learn which tools are best for certain effects.

Let us look at a general method of basic blow drying:

- Towel dry the hair after shampooing but do not remove too much water, if the hair is beginning to dry out it will not style properly. The water helps us get the shape because the hair becomes more supple when it is wet.

- Cleanly divide the hair into sections with clips. Use as many sections as you need to keep the hair under control and out of the way of the hair you are drying.

- For a one length bob take sections horizontally or diagonally, for a swept back look take vertical sections.

- Place the sectioned hair on to the brush with the thumb or fingers. When the hair is firmly on the brush direct the air from the dryer on to it. Move the brush down the section and the dryer with it. Repeat this process until the section is dried then move to the next section. Do this until all the hair has been dried. Hold the dryer at least 30cm away from the hair, any closer and the hair may be damaged.

- When we move the brush along the hair we do so in the direction we want the hair to go. When the hair is dried let it cool before combing or brushing all of the hair to blend all the hair together.

- If we want to get lift into the roots of the hair then we will lift the hair up and dry the root area first. Then we take the hair down and dry the lengths.

- If we want a curlier or casual effect then we use a roller brush and wind the hair around it and then dry. When we wind the brush out of the hair we leave it in the curl shape, wait until it is cool and then either brush or use a large toothed comb to blend the hair together to create the overall effect.

We can practise the different effects that different brushes have on a mannequin head. Try out your techniques and see what results you get.

> **REMEMBER** ✔
>
> Keep the drier moving and not too close to the hair and scalp, otherwise you may burn the scalp and damage the hair.

ACTIVITY 005–9

Find out:

1. Why you should check your dryer before use.

2. Why you must not use electrical equipment with wet hands.

3. Why you shouldn't blow dry hair that is in poor condition.

Make sure your tutor has checked your work. Tick when you have completed this activity.

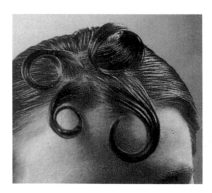

Different setting methods will give different types of curl

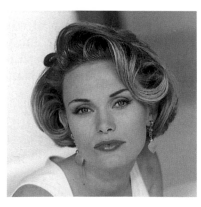

Dressing the curls gives a more structured look than the softer look of the blow dry

Some points to remember when you are blow drying:

- Check your dryer before you use it.
- Do not use electrical equipment with wet hands.
- Maintain a high standard of hygiene.
- Test the heat of the dryer before you use it.
- Direct hot air away from the scalp.
- Do not keep the dryer in one place too long.
- Use suitable drying aids, to help protect the hair.
- Do not blow dry hair that is in poor condition.

Setting the hair

Setting and dressing hair are important hairdressing techniques. Although not as popular as the blow drying techniques we have looked at, these techniques must be learned to allow us to achieve a wide range of effects that blow drying cannot.

Setting is the process of shaping wet hair, involving curling, rollering, twisting, pinning clipping and waving.

We are going to look at roller setting in this chapter. You will learn about the other techniques in level 2.

Dressing is the technique of blending the shapes we have created with the rollers, clips etc. into a finished style. This type of style tends to be more structured and formal than the softer casual look of the blow dry.

Roller setting

A method of styling the hair using 'rollers'. The hair is split into sections and then wound round the roller while it is wet. The scalp area is filled with rollers of different sizes in a variety of patterns. The pattern determines the shape of the style, while the size of the roller determines the amount of curl we put into the hair. If we use large rollers we will get soft curls; if we use small rollers we will get tight waves and curls.

Roller setting can be useful on fine hair as it will give an appearance of more hair because it usually creates more lift than blow drying.

Procedure for roller setting

Before we start we will have consulted with the client about the finished shape and decided on the size and pattern of the rollers.

- We start at the most convenient point.
- We section the hair into 'blocks' that are no wider or longer than the roller we are going to use. We do this using a tail comb.
- Next we comb the hair carefully and evenly up to a point, holding it away from us.

- Taking the roller, place the ends of the hair round the back of the roller so they appear over the top of the roller.
- Carefully, using the thumbs to hold the ends of the hair down, slowly wind the roller towards you. The ends should be in the middle of the roller and tucked under as you roll down. Continue to wind down till you reach the scalp. If you have rolled the hair correctly the roller should be on the root part of the section (not overhanging underneath).
- The roller is secured with a roller pin placed through and into the next roller. When all the rollers are in the hair a net is placed over them to keep them in place when the hair is dried.
- The client is then placed under a hood dryer and left for between 15 and 30 minutes, depending on the length and thickness of the hair.
- When the rollers have been removed the hair is dressed by brushing and combing into place.

Some points to remember when you are roller setting:

- Do not have the rollers too tight, remember the hair stretches when it is wet and goes back to its proper length as it dries.
- Do not put the securing pin into the roller so that it touches the scalp, they can be painful and if they are metal pins they can get hot and burn the scalp.
- The roller should sit on its own section. The hair should not fall off the ends of the roller.
- The ends of the hair must not be bent when the roller is put in.
- The hair must not be twisted.
- The hair should be allowed to cool when the client is removed from the dryer, then the rollers removed.
- Always use a bristle brush to brush the hair when roller setting, it is kinder to the hair and less painful to the client.

When dressing the hair.

- After the hair is dry and has been allowed to cool we remove the pins and the rollers.
- Using a soft bristle brush, brush the hair to loosen it and remove the roller marks.
- Next we brush the hair in the direction we want it and into the shape we want it.
- We then use a comb to finish the style.
- A light spray of hair spray to hold the hair in place will finish the dressing.

PLAITING AND BRAIDING

This is a method of finishing where we intertwine sections of hair. It can be an attractive way of dressing long hair. A variety of sizes and shapes is possible. The three stemmed plait is the most commonly used but we can use others. The use of additional materials and added hair is also popular. Here are some of the methods in use today:

ACTIVITY 005–10

Find some examples of the patterns of putting in rollers and the styles they will produce (these could be used in your assignment).

Make sure your tutor has checked your work. Tick when you have completed this activity.

REMEMBER ✔

Don't have your rollers too tight and don't let the securing pins touch the scalp.

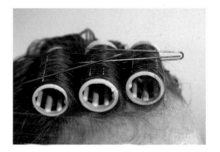

Securing rollers

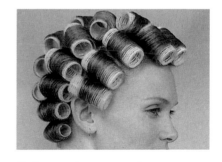

Roller setting: wound

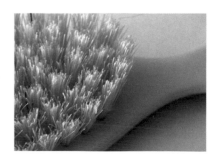

Soft bristle brush

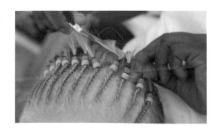

Cornrowing

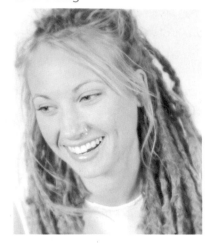

Dreadlocks

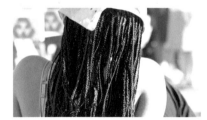

Hair wrapping

- Cornrowing. These are continuous plaits running along the scalp, sometimes called scalp plaits or ethnic plaits.
- Dreadlocks. These are long thin plaits often using added hair to increase the length.
- Hair wrapping. We use coloured ribbon to wrap around the hair or incorporate into a plait.
- Hair weaving. We interlace strands of hair over and under one another to produce a basketweave effect.

There is an infinite range of finishes that can be achieved with plaiting and braiding. A lot of the techniques have been imported from lots of ethnic groups around the world, particularly Africa.

Method for a French plait

When the shampoo is completed and the hair made ready the first steps in doing a French plait are as follows:

- Comb the front and top hair together at the crown and divide it into three equal stems.
- Starting from the left or right, cross an outside stem over the centre stem. Repeat this action, crossing the opposite stem over the centre stem.
- With the little finger take a further section of hair, about half the thickness of the original stem and add it to an outside stem.
- Cross this thickened stem over the centre stem and repeat this too, from the other outside stem.
- Continue in this way adding hair to each outside stem before crossing it over the centre stem.
- When there is no more hair to be added continue to plait to the ends of the hair and then secure the ends.

Good plaiting comes with practice. Make sure when you plait that you keep the right tension on the hair, to make sure you have it under control. Also make sure your hands follow the contours of the head so that the plait sits well along the back of the head.

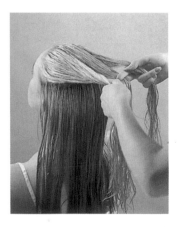

Sectioning the hair

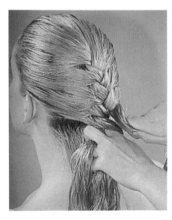

Plaiting the sections in with the main stem

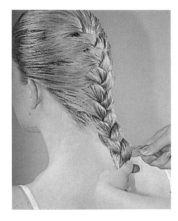

Continuing to plait

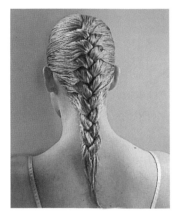

The completed plait

STYLING AIDS

We can use products to help us blow dry or set the hair. There is a huge range of products that we can choose from. Some will help the hair hold the shape we give it. Some will contain moisturisers to help condition the hair, others have shiners to give the hair a glossy sheen. Then there are waxes and gels that can be used to shape the hair after drying. We can use protectors to shield the hair from ultraviolet radiation. Hair spray is used after drying to hold the hair in place. It coats the hair with a fine plasticiser that breaks when we brush or comb the hair and is removed when we next wash the hair.

Try to learn about the styling aids that are available in your salon, it will improve the service you give to the clients.

ACTIVITY 005–11

Find out about the styling aids that are available in your salon and what they do and on what sort of hair they should be used.

Make sure your tutor has checked your work. Tick when you have completed this activity.

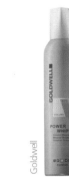
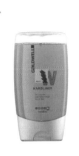
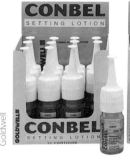
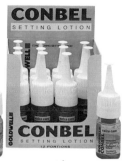

Goldwell

Goldwell

Goldwell

Styling products

CLIENT CONSULTATION SHEET

It is very important to keep records of what we do to our client's hair. It makes sure we can continue to keep out client's hair in the best condition. It also provides information about the treatments and services we have carried out on the client. Things like the products that were used, how they were used, processing times and most importantly the results. This means that we can repeat the successful processes at a later date with confidence. We could never remember all that information in our head.

Some salons will keep client record cards which record basic information, others will keep client consultation sheets which record all that was done on every visit. Many salons now keep this information on their salon computer system. One advantage of this is that all sorts of reports can be generated to help the salon.

We should complete a client consultation sheet with all the details of what we have done on each of our clients. It will help us develop our skills. To improve our skills we need to practise, the consultation sheets will tell us what we have not done much of and therefore need to do more of to make progress.

REMEMBER

Always complete a client consultation sheet for every client you do and keep them in your portfolio.

STYLES
SALON
HIGH STREET
LITTLE TOWN
LONDON
W1 1AD
020 12345
020 12345
styles@styles.co.uk
www.styles.co.uk

CUT
BLOW-DRY
SHAMPOO
SET
STRAIGHTENING
PERMS
COLOURS
HIGHLIGHTS
LOWLIGHTS
WEDDINGS
PARTIES
BEAUTY
TREATMENTS
MAKE-UP
MANICURES
VOUCHERS

CLIENT RECORD CARD			
NAME	ADDRESS		
TELEPHONE NUMBERS HOME WORK	DATE FIRST REGISTERED STYLIST	AGE GROUP	
HAIR CONDITION	SCALP	SKIN TYPE	

DATE	SERVICES AND PRODUCTS USED	REMARKS/PRICE CHARGED	STYLIST

A client record card

Key facts for you to remember from this chapter

- Keeping the salon clean will give the client a good impression of us.

- A clean salon will help prevent the transfer of infections and diseases.

- Dirty combs and brushes do not look good to the client.

- All the tools we use should be washed and/or sterilised after use.

- Make sure you prepare the client properly and protect all their clothing.

- Before we do anything to the client's hair we must make sure there are no problems that might prevent us from carrying out the service the client wants.

- Give the client a good shampoo and they will feel relaxed.

- Remember to make sure the client is seated comfortably at the back basin without any pressure on the back of their neck.

- Remember to rinse your hands thoroughly after shampooing and dry them carefully.

- Conditioners will smooth the cuticle making the hair shine and look good.

- Always remember to check your hair dryer before you use it.

- Make sure you fill in a client consultation sheet after every client.

GLOSSARY

Anti-bacterial   Ingredients in items like cleaners that help keep things free of bacteria.

Diffuser   An attachment that fits on to the end of a hand dryer that spreads the air over a wide area.

Nozzle   An attachment that fits on to the end of a hand dryer that concentrates the air flow in one direction.

Sterilisation   A process or material that kills all germs and leaves things sterile and germ free.

Ultraviolet radiation   These are rays that will kill bacteria. They are found in sunlight and from sunbeds.

Questions to test your knowlege of this unit

These are multiple-choice questions. Read the question carefully and then read the four possible answers. When you have decided which of the possible answers is the right one underline either a, b, c, or d in the box under the question.

1 Which of the following is a soft stroking movement used in shampooing?

a Rotary

b Effleurage

c Petrisage

d Friction

a	b	c	d

2 Large rollers used to set the hair will produce

a Waves

b Soft loose curls

c Strong tight curls

d Straight hair

a	b	c	d

3 Conditioners affect the cuticle layer by

a Hardening it

b Softening it

c Smoothing it

d Lifting it

a	b	c	d

4 A better shape will be achieved when we blow dry if the hair is

a Semi-dry

b Wet

c Saturated

d Coloured

a	b	c	d

5 Soft casual styles are achieved by

a Roller setting

b Blow drying

c Plaiting

d Dressing

a	b	c	d

Questions to test your knowlege of this unit (cont.)

Now try the following short answer questions. These may need a single word to answer or a short sentence or list.

1 Name three tools that would be used in the blow drying process and state what each does.

Answer 1. _____

2. _____

3. _____

2 Why do we use a gown and towels on the client?

Answer _____

_____

3 List three examples of plaiting.

Answer 1. _____

2. _____

3. _____

4 List three things that you should remember when you are blow drying.

Answer 1. _____

2. _____

3. _____

5 List two types of setting or blow drying aid we can use.

Answer 1. _____

2. _____

Helpful hints for the assignment

Introduction to the assignment

The assignment looks at what you have been learning about in this chapter: a variety of hair drying and braiding techniques.

Your tutor will give you the assignment and guide you on the maximum time you should allow to be sure of completing all of the course assignments.

Drying and plaiting techniques

For a style book showing examples of the effects that can be achieved when we use different techniques, you will need to find examples of hair that has been blow dried with a variety of brushes and using diffusers and nozzles. Also, examples of hair that has been finger dried and plaited or braided.

Trade magazines and hairdressing websites will provide you with good material. Manufacturers' advertising material is also useful. You can also use photographs of clients you have coloured in your practical work.

Pictures and presentation

When you have collected your material, think about presentation. Are you just going to stick the pictures on to paper or do you need to think about writing something to go with the pictures? If you think Yes, what information would be useful? Perhaps a description of the pictures, with what you think the effect of the drying technique is and some information about how it might have been carried out?

Next, think about how you are going to present your report. Decide whether you want to use a computer, or write it by hand. You should start with an introduction explaining what you are going to do, and what you are going to find out. Then add your information and pictures. Complete your report with some conclusions, and don't forget to include references (where your information came from).

Don't forget that presentation is important for this task.

CHECKERBOARD

After you have completed the chapter on Introduction to Hairdressing Services, rate yourself on the checkerboard. (You must be honest with yourself, don't put a tick in the box if you haven't done the work or don't feel that you have learned what you need to know.)

I understand why the work station needs to be prepared for the client ☐	I know how to prepare the client for hairdressing services ☐	I understand the importance of the consultation process ☐	I understand why things must be kept clean and sterilised before use ☐
I am aware of the methods of sterilisation used in the salon ☐	I can describe the basic structure of the hair and skin ☐	I understand why the hair is shampooed ☐	I know how to shampoo a client ☐
I know the massage movements used in shampooing and their effects ☐	I understand the purpose of conditioning the hair ☐	I am aware of the different types of conditioner and their effects on the hair ☐	I know how to condition the hair ☐
I understand what is meant by finishing techniques ☐	I know the tools required to achieve a blow dry ☐	I know how to carry out a basic blow dry ☐	I know the tools required to set the hair ☐
I can describe setting and dressing the hair ☐	I am aware of methods of plaiting and braiding ☐	I know how to carry out a basic plait ☐	I know how to complete a client consultation sheet ☐

ACTIVITY CHECKLIST

Make sure you have completed all the activities linked to this chapter and that you have put any information you need to keep in your portfolio.

Only tick the box and complete the portfolio reference when your tutor has confirmed the activity is complete.

	Complete	Portfolio Reference
Activity 005–1 (p. 72)	☐	
Activity 005–2 (p. 72)	☐	
Activity 005–3 (p. 73)	☐	
Activity 005–4 (p. 74)	☐	
Activity 005–5 (p. 75)	☐	
Activity 005–6 (p. 76)	☐	
Activity 005–7 (p. 77)	☐	
Activity 005–8 (p. 79)	☐	
Activity 005–9 (p. 82)	☐	
Activity 005–10 (p. 83)	☐	
Activity 005–11 (p. 85)	☐	

chapter 6

UNIT 006 INTRODUCTION TO BASIC PERMING AND COLOURING

Introduction

Two services that a client may want from their hairdresser is permanent waving (we usually call it perming) and hair colouring. Perming the hair will normally add curl to the hair so that we can style the hair differently or use the additional body that the perm process will give the hair. Colouring can be used for lots of reasons, for fashion using bright colours, to cover grey hair as we get older, or just because our client wants a change.

In this chapter we will introduce you to the basic skills of perming and the knowledge you will need to understand the perming process. We will also introduce you to the basics of colouring hair and the knowledge linking to it.

The main assessment requirement for this unit will be practical observations, where you will carry out the practical tasks we are going to look at in this chapter. There is also an assignment that you will complete. As a result of your practical work and the work we will do in this chapter, which will support your practical work, you will need to show that you are able to:

- **Prepare the work station to receive the client.**
- **Prepare the client for perming and colouring services.**
- **Assist in the consultation process.**
- **Select the products, tools and equipment required.**
- **Prepare the hair for the process.**
- **Carry out an element of the perming and colouring process.**
- **Prepare the hair for finishing services.**
- **Clear, clean and restore the work station.**

When we carry out our practical work, it is important at all times to follow all the things we learnt in Chapter 4 'Following Health and Safety Practice' and Chapter 1 'Finding out about Customer Service'. For example you should:

- **Demonstrate how to communicate in an effective professional manner with the clients.**

- **Ask appropriate questions to get any information you need from the client.**

- **Check equipment for faults and your work area for hazards.**

- **Follow procedures when using products.**

- **Record details on the client consultation sheet.**

- **Maintain a professional attitude.**

Remember your practical observations will be carried out by your tutor and, if you have completed the requirements of the statement, they will sign off the task. For the tasks in this unit you will be observed several times before your tutor will finally sign off all the tasks. You can gain a pass, credit or distinction in this element. Your tutor will explain what this means during your induction.

The assignment for this unit asks you to put together a small style book showing different results achieved using temporary and semi-permanent colours and perming.

WHAT YOU NEED TO KNOW

For the assignment which is part of the assessment for this unit you will need to:

- Find material that shows a range of effects achieved using perming, temporary and semi-permanent colours.
- Find out the actual process that was used to produce the effects in the examples.
- Find out what tools and equipment were used to produce the effects in the examples.

For the practical observation part of the assessment you will need to demonstrate, when you carry out your practical work, that you can:

- Get your work area ready for your client.
- Prepare your client for the initial part of the service.
- Identify the condition of the hair and scalp.
- Assist the stylist to decide the procedures required for the service.
- Get all your equipment and products ready.
- Carry out the practical element of the service (wind a minimum of ten **rods** and carry out a simulated neutralising for perming; apply, process and remove, if necessary, a colour under supervision for colouring).

- Prepare the client for the finishing service.
- Complete the consultation sheet and client record.
- Clean the work station.

Remember the observation can gain you a pass, credit or distinction.

This chapter will help you understand what you are learning in your practical work. When you have completed it you should:

- Understand the purpose of perming.
- Have a basic knowledge of the changes that take place in the hair during the perming process.
- Be able to describe the process of winding rods and how to avoid undesirable effects.
- Know the equipment, tools and materials required to prepare the client and work station.
- Be able to state why extra protection for the client is required when perming.
- Know how to clean and sterilise equipment and the work station.
- Be able to describe the 'neutralising' process.
- Understand the purpose of colouring the hair.
- Have a basic knowledge of the changes that take place in the hair during the colouring process.
- Know the methods of application used for temporary and semi-permanent colours.
- Know the equipment, tools and materials required to prepare the client and work station.
- Know how to remove excess colour material and when processing is complete.
- Know how to clear, clean and restore the work station.

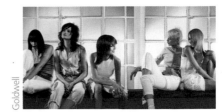

Perming and colouring

PERMANENT WAVING

We mostly use the word perming to describe the process of permanently adding curl to the hair. The process is highly technical and requires a great deal of knowledge and experience to carry out. Perming is always done by an experienced stylist.

In the first part of this chapter we will look at the basics of perming so you will understand how it works.

The shape of the hair is changed by using a chemical that alters the structure of the hair to a new shape and then another chemical to fix that new shape permanently. We wind the hair around rods of different sizes to determine what the new shape will be.

This process is very complex but it can be described very simply by imagining the hair is like a ladder. The long sides of the ladder are the parts of the hair that run along its length and the rungs of the ladder are the parts that hold the hair together.

KEY FACT

Perming is the process of adding curl to the hair permanently.

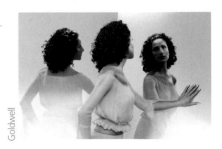

Permanent waving

KEY FACT

The perming solution can cause serious burns to the skin or eyes if it is misused. *Always* use it with care and follow the instructions.

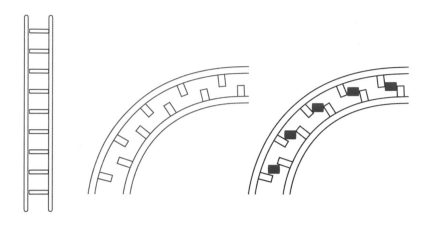

The ladder analogy

When the **perming solution** is applied to the hair it will work to partly breakdown the hair structure. In our ladder it would look as if we had sawn the rungs in half. Remember the hair would be wound round the rod so the rungs would move away from each other as you can see in the diagram.

When we use the **neutraliser** this makes the rungs join up again but in the new position not the original one. The neutralising process is important because if we do not do it right the hair will not be fixed in the new shape so will go back to a straighter shape.

Like all hairdressing processes the service begins with getting the client ready for the service. So the first thing we need to do is as follows.

Prepare the work station

In Chapter 5, Unit 005 Introduction to hairdressing services we learnt how the work station should be made ready for the client. Here is a reminder.

When the client is moved from the reception to our work station it is important that it is clean and tidy. We must make sure that:

- The floor area is clean and free from hair or anything else.
- The chair is clean.
- The mirror is clean with no smudges or dirty patches.
- If there is a shelf it is clean and tidy.
- The trolley is also clean and tidy and everything in it proper place.

Remember, make sure the client gets the right impression when they are brought to the salon floor. A clean work area shows a care and pride in your work.

Preparing the client

When we have seated the client, we prepare them as we did in Chapter 5. Here is a reminder. We need a gown, towels and perhaps tissues or cotton wool.

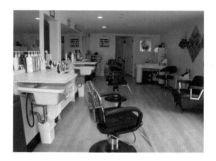

Remember the salon needs to be clean, tidy and safe to give the right impression

REMEMBER ✔

If you do not have anything to do then clean and tidy anything that needs it. Teamwork and helping colleagues is important.

ACTIVITY 006–1

Find out more about why we have to protect the client's clothes and property when they are in the salon.

Make sure your tutor has checked your work. Tick when you have completed this activity.

The fresh clean gown is placed over the client to cover their clothes. A clean towel is then placed round their neck and across their shoulders and the tissue or cotton wool is put around the neck.

Client consultation

The stylist will discuss with the client their requirements and make a number of decisions about the perming process. These decisions are very important if the process is going to be successful. They will range from the size and pattern of the rods to be used to the type of shampoo to be used. This process will use chemicals and so the condition of the hair and scalp has to be carefully assessed so that there is no danger to the client. We should remind ourselves of this process by re-reading the relevant part of Chapter 5.

When the consultation is complete we can then carry out the service.

Carrying out a perm

For most perms the hair is shampooed before we do the perm. We would use a shampoo that contained no additives which might be left on the hair and interfere with the chemical process. The shampoo would be carried out as described in Chapter 5. After the hair is combed additional protection will be used. A waterproof gown will be used or a waterproof shoulder cape, plus another towel over the shoulders. This is because we are using chemicals on the hair which could damage the client's clothes.

The next part of the process is to divide the hair into sections according to the type of perm we want to do. For a basic perm the hair would be divided into nine sections. We make the sections with the **tail comb**. The section should be about 5cm wide just less than the length of the rod (use the rod as a guide). The sections are secured with long clips (these are sometimes called sectioning clips).

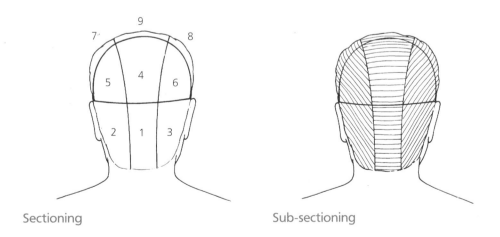

Sectioning   Sub-sectioning

We are now ready to wind in the rods. To do this we will:

- Divide the sections we have made into smaller ones as we wind in the rods. The section of hair should not be wider or longer than the rod we are using.

KEY FACT

All the decisions for a perm are vital to getting a good result. If one decision is wrong then the stylist could struggle to get a good result.

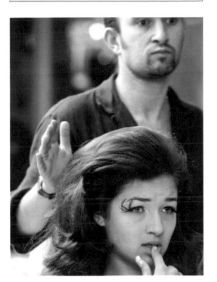

Client consultation

REMEMBER

The section must be neat and even, it helps you wind properly and looks professional to the client.

ACTIVITY 006–2

Find out more about rod sizes and the colour code for them.

Make sure your tutor has checked your work. Tick when you have completed this activity.

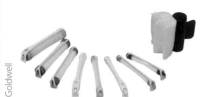

REMEMBER

One rod put in wrongly can ruin the perm and the client's hair.

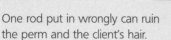

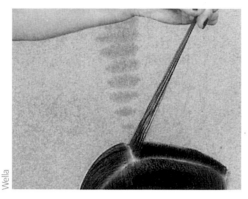

Perming curlers

- Using your comb, comb the hair away from you and make the ends of the hair into a flat point in the middle of the section.
- Put an '**end paper**' (a piece of tissue used to wrap round the ends of the hair) round the ends
- Select the correct rod size and wind the rod down from the ends to the roots (the part of the hair nearest the scalp).
- Secure the rod with the elastic strap.
- Repeat the process for all the section and then all the sections.

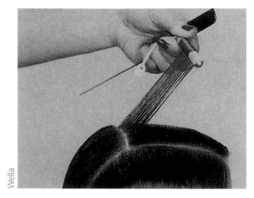

Winding: taking a hair section

Winding the section on to the curler

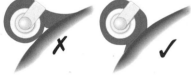

Winding: depth of section

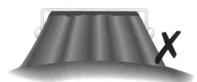

Winding: width of section

Winding a perm rod

It is very important that when we wind a rod into the hair, when we are perming, we do so properly. If we make mistakes we must remember that mistakes could be permanent. Always make sure when you wind the rod that:

- The section is the correct size.
- The hair is combed evenly.
- The ends of the hair are not bent or twisted under the end wrap.
- The rod is wound evenly down to the scalp.
- The hair is not pulled too tight when the rod is secured.
- The elastic strap is not pressing on the hair at the ends of the rods.
- The rod sits across the middle of its section.
- You check every rod before processing.

When all the hair is wound then the perming solution will be applied, the perm will now be allowed to process. When we do this we must use rubber gloves (remember PPE from Health and Safety). When this is complete we must neutralise the perm.

This part of the perm is usually part of the junior's duties.

The first thing to do is to take the client to a basin and sit them comfortably.

- Turn on the water and test the temperature (use slightly cooler water as the scalp may be more sensitive from the previous work).

- Rinse the hair thoroughly for approximately 3 minutes. We must make sure that all the curlers are thoroughly rinsed to remove the excess perm solution so that it stops working. (If it were left on the hair it could do very serious damage to the hair even breaking it.)

- Using a towel blot the curlers carefully to remove as much excess moisture as you can.

- Next we mix the neutraliser according to the manufacturer's instructions.

- Apply about half of the neutraliser to the hair and make sure all the rods are covered. A piece of cotton wool can be placed round the hairline to stop the neutraliser running down the client's face. Keep the rest of the neutraliser for later.

- We now leave the neutraliser on the hair for a period of time, this is usually 5 minutes but may vary according to the instructions.

- Then we very carefully undo the elastic straps on the rods and wind the rods out of the hair (we must not pull the hair because the fixing process is not complete).

- Next apply the rest of the neutraliser to the ends of the hair and leave for another 5 minutes or for as long as the instructions say.

- Lastly rinse thoroughly to remove all traces of the neutraliser.

The client can now be moved to the work station for their finishing service.

We must not forget to clear, clean and restore the basin area, ready for another client.

As you progress your career to level 2 you will learn more about the perming process and develop your skills to be able to carry out the complete perming process.

COLOURING THE HAIR

People have been colouring their hair for at least 2,500 years. The ancient Egyptians used **henna** to colour their hair. Henna is made from a plant and colours the hair red.

Nowadays we have a huge range of products available to change the colour of the hair. Some change the colour permanently, some temporarily, between shampoos or for a number of shampoos. The range of colours we can achieve is also huge, virtually everything but pure white. We should remember here that we cannot achieve any colour on any client. The colouring process works in several ways:

- Adding colour pigments to the hair to enhance the hair's natural colour, these are usually called temporary, or semi-permanent colours.

- Removing the hair's natural pigment and replacing it with artificial pigment, these are usually called permanent colours.

ACTIVITY 006-3

Find out what the chemical is that fixes the hair in the new position.

Make sure your tutor has checked your work. Tick when you have completed this activity.

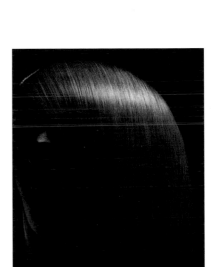

Goldwell

Coloured hair

ACTIVITY 006-4

Find out the name of the natural pigment found in hair.

Make sure your tutor has checked your work. Tick when you have completed this activity.

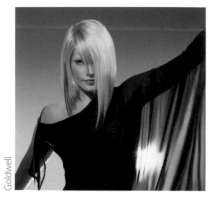

Goldwell

Bleached hair

● Just removing the hair's natural pigment, this process is usually called bleaching.

Like perming, colouring is a complex technique that requires a great deal of knowledge, skill and understanding. Most colouring is carried out by the stylists. Some parts of the process are often carried out by the junior staff, applying the colour to the hair and removing it when it has processed are the main ones.

The most difficult part of the colouring process is selecting the colour to use to achieve what the client wants. It is not as simple as looking at the paint chart to find a colour to decorate a room. When you progress to level 2 you will begin to learn about colour selection and develop your practical skills.

In this part of the chapter we will look at how we use temporary and semi-permanent colours.

Temporary colours

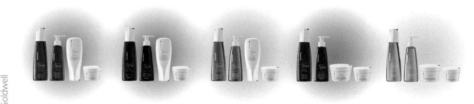

Goldwell

Temporary colour products

> **REMEMBER** ✔
>
> You cannot lighten the colour of the hair with temporary colours.

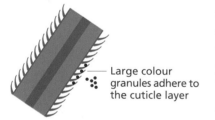

Large colour granules adhere to the cuticle layer

> **ACTIVITY 006–5**
>
> Make a list of the temporary colours that are used in the salon and the colours they are available in.
>
> Make sure your tutor has checked your work. Tick when you have completed this activity.
>
>

Temporary colours will add colour to the client's natural colour to improve it. For example we can add some red pigment to make the hair look brighter and warmer, or if the client's hair is naturally red we can add an ash shade to cool it down and make it look less red. We can use bright colours on parts of the hair to make it show up. Temporary colours come in a range of types:

● Gel
● **Mousse**
● Water rinses
● Coloured hair spray
● Glitter and colour spray
● Colour paints
● Colour setting aid

Some of these colours are applied to wet hair others to dry hair. They work by sticking to the cuticle scale of the hair.

Gel, mousse, water rinses and coloured setting aid are usually applied to wet hair after shampooing is completed and just before the finishing service is started. Coloured hair spray, coloured paints and glitter and colour spray are usually applied to the hair after finishing services have been given. The advantages of temporary colours are:

- The colour effect is only temporary.
- A wide range of colours is available.
- The colourant is easily removed by washing.
- The condition of the hair can be improved.
- Subtle tones can be added to white and grey hair.
- Fashion effects can be achieved on bleached hair.
- They do not usually cause problems with the skin.

The disadvantages are:

- They cannot be used to lighten the hair.
- They can be patchy on hair that is damaged or in poor condition.
- Results can be patchy on hair with quantities of grey hair.

Application of a temporary colour

The application of the gel, mousse or water rinse will start after the hair has been shampooed (Chapter 5 will remind you of the procedure p. 78).

The stylist will have decided the type and shade of colour that will give the client the result they want during the consultation. It is important if we are going to use the gel, mousse, water-based or coloured setting aid that all traces of previously used product have been removed when the hair is shampooed (as these might prevent the colour from sticking to the hair and make the result patchy).

- Towel dry the hair well to remove excess moisture. If the hair is too wet it will dilute the colour and it could run down the client's neck and face.
- Use a plastic shoulder cape or special colour gown to cover the client's clothes and a black towel around their shoulders (salons will use black towels for colours to give extra protection against damage to the client's clothes).
- Apply the colour to the hair using a sponge or brush or direct from the container.
- Comb the hair away from the face.
- Brush or sponge the colour on to the hair from front to back.
- If the colour is being used direct from the container gently pour the colour on to the hair again from the front to the back.
- Make sure the colour does not run on to the face.
- Use a gentle rotary movement of the fingers to distribute the colour through the hair, or carefully comb the hair. Combing can be useful on longer hair.
- If the hair is long then we can section the hair to keep it under control.

When the application is complete we can begin the drying process we have selected.

Remember to protect your hands from staining by wearing gloves if necessary.

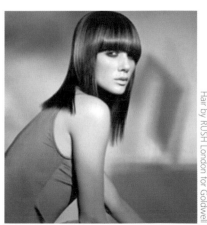

Coloured hair

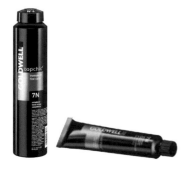

Goldwell

Colouring products

> **REMEMBER** ✔
>
> Semi-permanent colours will last between six and eight shampoos.

> **REMEMBER** ✔
>
> Semi-permanent colours will not lighten the hair.

> **ACTIVITY 006–6**
>
> Make a list of the semi-permanent colours that are used in the salon and the colours they are available in.
>
> Make sure your tutor has checked your work. Tick when you have completed this activity.
>
> ☐

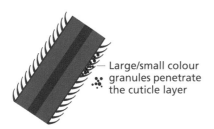

Large/small colour granules penetrate the cuticle layer

> **REMEMBER** ✔
>
> Semi-permanent colours can stain the skin. Be careful when you apply them, try not to put colour on the skin outside the hairline.

Semi-permanent colours

Semi-permanent colours are used to enhance the natural colour of a client's hair for a short period of time. Most will gradually fade from the hair each time the hair is washed, this can be between six and eight shampoos. Like temporary colours they are used to add colour to the client's natural colour to enhance and enrich it. There is a good range of colours but we must be careful to make the right selection.

Semi-permanent colours work by penetrating the cuticle layer and laying between the cuticle and the cortex (remember the hair structure from Chapter 5), from where they are gradually removed by washing. This is what makes them last longer.

Semi-permanent colours are available in different types, for example, mousse in aerosol cans, gels and creams. Most are ready to use and do not require any mixing. Always check the manufacturer's instructions to make sure.

Semi-permanent colours have to be left on the hair for a period of time for them to work. This is called the 'processing' time. Some ranges of colour have to be heated under a dryer or steamer, the instructions will explain what needs to be done.

The advantages of semi-permanent colours are:

- They are more effective and longer lasting than temporary colours.
- They are available in a larger range of colours.
- There is no regrowth, unless the hair is porous, as the colour is removed by the time the hair has grown.
- Natural colour is not affected.
- They do not usually cause skin problems (check the manufacturer's instructions).

The disadvantages are:

- The hair colour cannot be made lighter using these colours.
- They can last a long time if the hair is porous.
- They do not work well on hair with a high percentage of grey/white.

Application of a semi-permanent colour

As we saw with temporary colours the stylist would consult with the client and decide on the type and shade of colour that would be used on the client. The stylist will also have checked the scalp carefully to make sure there are no cuts, **abrasions** or other things that might be aggravated by the chemical in the colour.

The next stage will be to prepare the client for the colour application. Some semi-permanent colours do not require the hair to washed before application, you will find this out from the instructions and the stylist will confirm what they want you to do. This type of colour usually has detergent in it which will clean the hair when the colour is removed.

The next thing to do will be to prepare the client for the colour:

- Either dampen the hair with warm water or shampoo the hair in the normal way, according to the manufacturer's instructions.
- Towel dry to remove excess water.
- Place a colour gown on the client, this is waterproof and will make sure that colour cannot get through to the client's clothes.
- Black or special colour towels are used around the shoulders.
- Comb the hair through to remove tangles.
- Apply the colour using a sponge, brush, applicator bottle or direct from the container, according to the manufacturer's instructions.
- The hair can be sectioned into four with a parting from the forehead to the nape in the middle of the head and then from ear to ear over the crown. Each section can be secured with a clip.
- Starting with one of the sections, divide that into smaller sections brushing or sponging colour on to the hair as you go.
- Repeat this for the other three sections so that all the hair is covered.
- Be careful not to put colour on to the skin outside the hairline as it may stain temporarily. If you do then wipe carefully with a little damp cotton wool.
- Leave the colour to process following the manufacturer's instructions.
- Remove the excess colour by rinsing as instructed by the manufacturer.

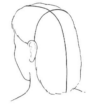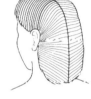

Hair sectioning

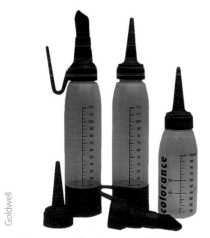

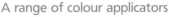
Goldwell

A range of colour applicators

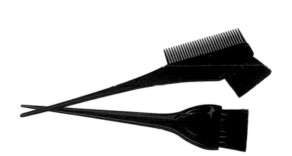

Mahogany Hairdressing (www.mahogany.co.uk)

Applying colour

CLIENT CONSULTATION SHEET

It is very important to keep detailed records of the colouring and perming process that we carried out on our client. It makes sure we can continue to keep our client's hair in the best condition. Details of the products that were used, how they were used, processing times and, most importantly, the results should be recorded. This means that we can repeat the successful processes at a later date with confidence. We could never remember all that information in our head.

REMEMBER

Always complete a client consultation sheet for every client you do and keep them in your portfolio.

Some salons will keep client record cards, which record basic information, others will keep client consultation sheets, which record all that was done on every visit. Many salons now keep this information on their salon computer system. One advantage of this is that all sorts of reports can be generated to help the salon.

We should complete a client consultation sheet with all the details of what we have done on each of our clients. It will help us develop our skills. To improve our skills we need to practice, the consultation sheets will tell us what we have not done much of and therefore need to do more of to make progress.

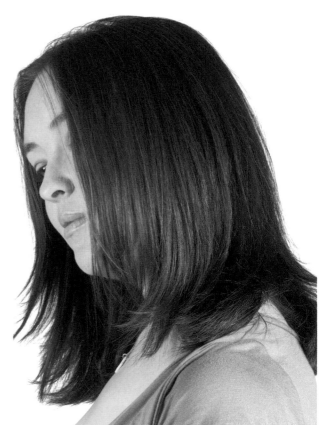

Colour can create a range of different looks for your client and transform any cut

Key facts for you to remember from this chapter

- Permanent waving changes the shape of the hair by altering the hair structure using a chemical.
- Extra protection is needed for the client's clothes etc.
- Only use shampoo made for use before perming, some are called pre-perm shampoos.
- Every perm rod must be put into the hair correctly, mistakes can be permanent.
- The neutralising process must be carried out correctly to ensure the curl we want in the hair is 'fixed'.
- Clients colour their hair to enhance the colour, cover grey or white hair and for fashion.
- Extra protection is needed for the client's clothes etc.
- Temporary colours last between shampoos and are easily washed out of the hair.
- Semi-permanent colour lasts for between six and eight shampoos.

GLOSSARY

Abrasions   An injury to the skin where lots of tiny cuts are found on the surface, usually as the result of grazing the skin against a rough surface.

End paper   A piece of tissue that is used to wrap the ends of the hair when we wind in the rods.

Henna   A vegetable hair colour made from a plant called *lawsonia inermis*, a member of the privet family. Used in ancient Egypt and today.

Mousse   This is a term used to describe products that have the consistency of thick creamy froth, the products are mainly colour and setting aids.

Neutralising   The process that makes the curl we have achieved with the perming solution and rods permanent.

Perming solution   The chemical that changes the structure of the hair.

Rods   The curlers that we wind into the hair in the perming process. They come in different sizes and are sometimes colour coded.

Tail comb   A comb with fine teeth one end and a pointed spike at the other, used for combing the hair and taking sections of the hair.

Questions to test your knowlege of this unit

These are multiple-choice questions. Read the question carefully and then read the four possible answers. When you have decided which of the possible answers is the right one underline either a, b, c, or d in the box under the question.

1 When perm solution is applied to the hair it will

   a heat the hair

   b break down the structure

   c melt the hair

   d wet the hair

a	b	c	d

2 For a basic permanent wave the hair is usually divided into

   a 5 sections

   b 7 sections

   c 9 sections

   d 11 sections

a	b	c	d

3 Temporary colours will stick to the

   a Cortex

   b Cuticle

   c Medulla

   d Follicle

a	b	c	d

4 Semi-permanent colours will last

   a 6 to 8 washes

   b 4 to 6 washes

   c up to 9 washes

   d up to 12 washes

a	b	c	d

5 How many sections should the hair be divided into for the application of a semi-permanent colour?

   a 2

   b 4

   c 6

   d 8

a	b	c	d

Questions to test your knowlege of this unit (cont.)

Now try the following short answer questions. These may need a single word to answer or a short sentence or list.

1 Semi-permanent colour can lighten the client's natural colour – True or False?

Answer _____

_____

2 What size should the section be for a perm rod?

Answer _____

_____

3 What sort of gown should you use on the client when applying a semi-permanent colour?

Answer _____

_____

4 Describe briefly what neutralising does to the hair during a permanent wave.

Answer _____

_____

5 Give three advantages of a semi-permanent colour.

Answer   1. _____

2. _____

3. _____

Helpful hints for the assignment

Introduction to the assignment

The assignment looks at what you have been learning about in this chapter: the looks that can be achieved with temporary or semi-permanent colours and perming techniques.

Your tutor will give you the assignment and guide you on the maximum time you should allow to be sure of completing all of the course assignments.

Perms, temporary and semi-permanent colours

For a style book showing examples of the effects that can be achieved when we use perms, temporary and semi-permanent colours, you will need to find examples of hair that has been permed and coloured with temporary and semi permanent colours. Trade magazines and hairdressing websites will provide you with good material. Manufacturers' advertising material is also useful. You can also use photographs of clients you have coloured in your practical work.

Pictures and presentation

When you have collected your material, think about presentation. Are you just going to stick the pictures on to paper or do you need to think about writing something to go with the pictures? If you think Yes, what information would be useful? Perhaps a description of the pictures, with what you think the effect of the perm or colour is and some information about how it might have been carried out?

Next, think about how you are going to present your report. Decide whether you want to use a computer, or write it by hand. You should start with an introduction, this explains what you are going to do, and what you are going to find out. Then add your information and pictures. Complete your report with some conclusions, and don't forget to include references (where your information came from).

Don't forget that presentation is important for this task.

CHECKERBOARD

After you have completed the chapter on Introduction to Basic Perming and Colouring, rate yourself on the checkerboard. (You must be honest with yourself, don't put a tick in the box if you haven't done the work or don't feel that you have learned what you need to know.)

I understand what the perming process is ☐	I have a basic understanding of what happens to the hair during the perming process ☐	I am aware of things that would cause a client to stop coming to the salon ☐	I know how to prepare the client for the perming process ☐
I know the procedure for sectioning the hair and winding the perm rods ☐	I understand the process of neutralising the perm ☐	I can section and wind ten perm rods on a client ☐	I can carry out the process of neutralising a perm ☐
I understand what temporary colours are and how they work ☐	I can describe the advantages and disadvantages of temporary colours ☐	I know the process of applying temporary colours to the hair ☐	I can apply a temporary colour to a client's hair ☐
I understand how semi-permanent colours work ☐	I can describe the advantages and disadvantages of semi-permanent colours ☐	I know the process of applying a semi-permanent colour to a client's hair ☐	I can apply a semi-permanent colour to a client's hair ☐

CHECKER BOARD ✓

ACTIVITY CHECKLIST

Make sure you have completed all the activities linked to this chapter and that you have put any information you need to keep in your portfolio.

Only tick the box and complete the portfolio reference when your tutor has confirmed the activity is complete.

	Complete	Portfolio Reference
Activity 006–1 (p. 96)	☐	
Activity 006–2 (p. 97)	☐	
Activity 006–3 (p. 99)	☐	
Activity 006–4 (p. 99)	☐	
Activity 006–5 (p. 100)	☐	
Activity 006–6 (p. 102)	☐	

chapter 7

UNIT 007 APPLYING BASIC MAKE-UP

Introduction

In this chapter we are going to cover the skills and knowledge you will need to prepare the client, set up the working area and carry out a basic make-up treatment.

The main assessment requirement for this unit will be practical observations, where you will carry out the practical tasks we are going to look at in this chapter. There is also an assignment that you will complete. As a result of your practical work and the work we will do in this chapter you will need to show you are able to:

- **Prepare your work area.**
- **Prepare your client for the treatment.**
- **Carry out a consultation and complete a treatment plan.**
- **Carry out a basic make-up.**
- **Recognise basic skin structure.**
- **State the functions of the skin.**
- **List the conditions which may prevent or restrict treatments.**
- **Outline reactions which may occur and how you would deal with them.**
- **Understand how to use the products and equipment needed to carry out a make-up.**

When we carry out a basic make-up treatment, it is important at all times to follow all the things we learnt in Chapter 4 'Following Health and Safety Practice' and Chapter 1 'Finding out about Customer Service'.

Remember your practical observations will be carried out by your tutor and, if you have completed the requirements of the observation criteria, they will sign off the task. For the tasks in this unit you will be observed several times before your tutor will finally sign off all tasks. You can gain a pass, credit or distinction in this element. Your tutor will explain what this means during your induction.

WHAT YOU NEED TO KNOW

To complete the assignment for this unit you will need to:

- Find out about the current and emerging trends in the use of make-up.
- Find examples of a range of make-ups for day, evening, fantasy and for brides.
- Find out the type of make-up products and design techniques that might be used for your examples.

During the practical observation you will need to demonstrate that you can:

- Prepare your work area ready for your client.
- Have all your equipment ready to use.
- Carry out a consultation and complete a treatment plan.
- Prepare the skin for a basic make-up treatment.
- Carry out a basic make-up.
- Use face paints to create a desired effect.
- Discuss the aftercare advice with your client.
- Clear away your tools and products.
- Clean your work area.

Remember the observation can gain you a pass, credit or distinction.

MAKE-UP

We use make-up for a variety of reasons, these include:

- To enhance natural features.
- To disguise or soften features.
- To conceal blemishes.

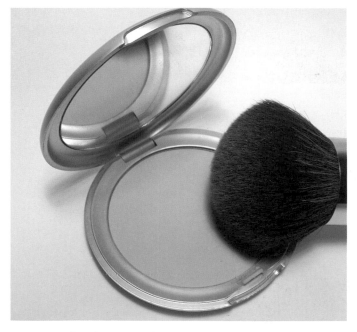
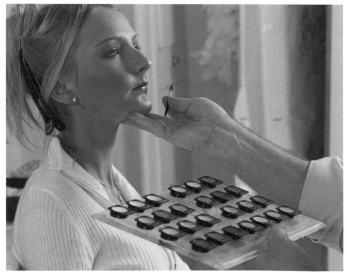

An example of some make-up products

- To create a dramatic effect.
- To create a decorative effect.
- To improve skin condition.

Using make-up helps the client feel more confident about themselves. Each client is unique, so each treatment needs to be tailored to their needs. It needs to complement their personality and lifestyle and suit the occasion the make-up will be seen in.

Those occasions may include:

- A day make-up for general wear, including work.
- An evening make-up for an evening out or special occasion.
- A theatrical/fantasy make-up for a party or similar occasion.

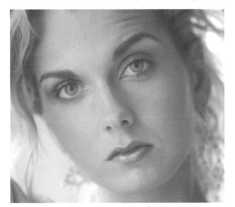 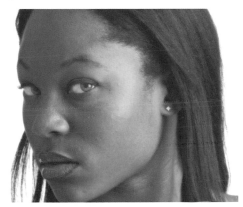

Day make-up

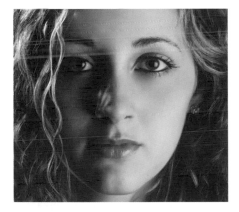 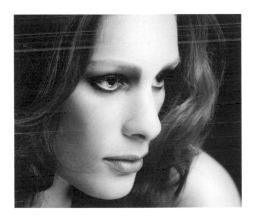

Evening make-up

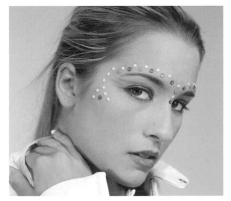 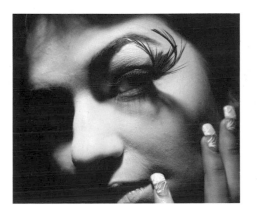

Fantasy make-up

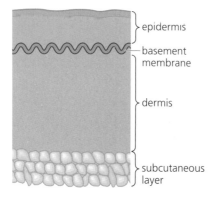

epidermis

basement membrane

dermis

subcutaneous layer

Skin

ACTIVITY 007–1

Find out more about the structure of the epidermis. Look at the different layers of the epidermis and how the layers are formed.

Make sure your tutor has checked your work. Tick when you have completed this activity.

KEY FACT !

When we cleanse the skin we remove dead skin cells from the epidermis.

ACTIVITY 007–2

Find out more about the structure of the dermis. Look at the different things that are contained in it.

Make sure your tutor has checked your work. Tick when you have completed this activity.

REMEMBER ✓

The word SHAPES will remind you of the basic functions of the skin.

ANATOMY AND PHYSIOLOGY

To become a successful beauty therapist we must know a lot about the body and how it works. Later in your career you will learn about the muscles, nerves and systems like the blood supply. For this course we need to learn about the skin, how it works and functions and in the next chapter we learn about the nails.

The skin

The skin is the largest organ in the body and it is very important for us to know about it, particularly when we are working on the face. The skin varies in appearance, according to our race, sex and age. It also changes from season to season, and from year to year. It can be affected by how we treat it, the medication we take and what we eat.

We need to know its basic structure and function so we can improve its appearance and understand how to care for it. The skin types and conditions of the skin depend on the functioning of different parts of the skin. We will look at the skin types and conditions later on in this chapter.

The basic structure of the skin

The top two layers of the skin are called the:

- Epidermis
- Dermis

The **epidermis** is the top or outer layer of the skin. Its main function is to protect the body from what goes around it. The epidermis is mostly formed from dead cells that are being rubbed off. We lose millions of dead skin cells from the top of the epidermis every day.

The **dermis** lies underneath the epidermis and is much thicker. It is sometimes called the 'living skin' because it is made up of living functioning cells. The dermis contains lots of different structures, including all the nerve endings, the sebaceous glands, the sweat glands and a blood supply. When you massage the surface of the skin you increase the blood supply, which helps to improve the health and function of the skin.

Basic functions of the skin

Although one of the skin's functions is to **protect** there are lots of other important functions and they all need to be remembered.

There are six functions:

- **Sensation**
- **Heat regulation**
- **Absorption**
- **Protection**
- **Excretion**
- **Secretion**

Skin types

Even though we now know the structure of the skin and its functions, before we can carry out any treatment on the skin we need to learn about skin types. The type of skin our client has will affect how we carry out the treatment, what we use and in some cases what precautions we take. There are four basic skin types:

1 Dry skin

2 Oily skin

3 Combination skin

4 Normal skin

How to recognise skin types

Dry skin

Dry skin lacks oil, moisture or both. A dry skin:

- Has small tight pores.
- Has poor moisture content.
- Has a thin and coarse texture.
- Has flaky patches of skin.
- Can be sensitive.
- Can age quicker.

Oily skin

Oily skin produces more oil than a normal skin. An oily skin:

- Has large pores.
- Appears thick and coarse.
- Appears shiny.
- May have blackheads and spots present.

Combination skin

Combination skin can be partly dry and partly oily. The oily part is often known as the T-zone, this is often on the forehead, nose and chin. The rest of the face is dry. A combination skin has:

- Large pores in the T-zone, but small pores in the dry areas.
- Coarse and thick skin on the T-zone, but thin coarse skin on the dry areas.
- Blackheads and spots may be present in the T-zone and the cheek areas can look sensitive.

ACTIVITY 007–3

Find out more about the six functions of the skin. List the functions, explain what they are.

Make sure your tutor has checked your work. Tick when you have completed this activity.

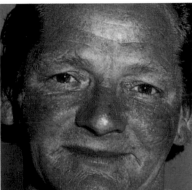

Dry skin

Dr Gray, The World of Skin Care

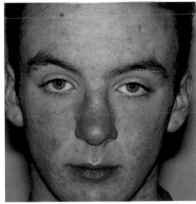

Oily skin

Dr Gray, The World of Skin Care

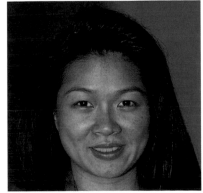

Combination skin

Dr Gray, The World of Skin Care

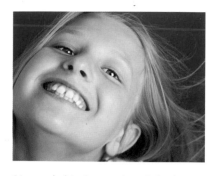

Normal skin is rare in adults but is often seen in pre-pubescent children

Normal skin

Normal skin can also be called balanced skin, because it is neither too oily nor too dry. Normal skin in adults is rare; it can often be seen in young pre-puberty skin. Normal skin has:

- Small or medium size pores.
- Good moisture content.
- A skin texture that is even and smooth.
- A colour that is healthy.

ACTIVITY 007–4

Find out if you can recognise different skin types from the information above. Look at each other's skin and see if you can decide what skin type each of you have.

Make sure your tutor has checked your work. Tick when you have completed this activity.

A BASIC MAKE-UP

Preparing the work area

KEY FACT

Keeping the salon clean will reduce the risk of transferring infections and diseases. It will also give the right impression to the client.

REMEMBER

If you drop any make-up tools on the floor do not use them on the client's skin. To avoid cross infection all equipment must be cleaned before and after use.

There are lots of things we must consider in the preparation of our working area and for the treatment itself. A make-up treatment consist of three main stages:

1 Preparing the skin, by cleansing, toning and moisturising.
2 Applying the make-up in a set sequence.
3 Giving aftercare advice.

For our work area we need to think about the health and safety precautions involved:

- Is the floor area clean and free from spillages or anything else?
- Is the chair and work surface clean?
- If there is a trolley is it clean and tidy?
- Is the equipment to hand?

Remember our work on impressions in Chapters 1 and 2, make sure the client gets the right impression when they are brought to the salon or work area. A clean work area shows you take care and pride in your work.

Carrying out a basic make-up treatment involves sanitising the work area and using tools and products which can be disposed of or cleaned quite easily.

The work area must be wiped over with a sanitising solution before and after treatment.

- Once the work surface has been **sanitised** the products may be displayed for the client to see.
- Make sure your brushes are clean and dry.
- Have your make-up palette clean and ready to use.
- Make sure the cleansing products are within reach.
- A mirror should be available if the client is not placed in front of a make-up mirror.
- The room should be well lit.
- A lined bin should be placed beside the working area.
- Position a stool or chair for yourself and the client.
- A clean gown and head band should be used on the client to protect their hair and clothes.

There are some other points we must consider when setting up and selecting our tools, equipment and products. The chart below includes the products, tools and equipment we may need and health and safety factors that need to be followed.

Product	Use	Health and safety
Sanitising solution Ellisons	To wipe over work area and surfaces. Sanitising liquid prevents the multiplication of micro-organisms, but it does not kill all micro-organisms	Could cause a slippage if spilt. Might cause skin irritation and could be toxic if swallowed. Chemical sterilising sprays are also used to sanitise the surface of the work area. These should be used following manufacturer's instructions and in a well ventilated area. Avoid contact with flame and excessive heat
Make-up brushes Ellisons	To apply make-up	Clean before and after use with a detergent, disinfectant and sanitising solution. Rinse well and dry thoroughly
Make-up applicators 	Usually sponge applicators. May be disposable to prevent cross infection	Use disposable applicator if possible to prevent cross infection, in particular mascara wands
Orange sticks Ellisons	Disposable wooden tools, usually with a hoof shape at one end and pointed the other. They can be used to remove product from containers	Never reuse the orange stick, throw away after each treatment to avoid cross infection. Always tip with clean cotton wool if using on the skin
Cosmetic sponges Ellisons	To use in the application of foundation. If a light application of foundation is required it is advisable to damp the sponge	These sponges must be washed out in hot soapy water to remove all traces of make-up. The sponges should never be dipped into a jar or pot of foundation

Product		Use	Health and safety
Cleanser		A cleansing product helps remove all traces of dirt, grime and old make-up	Tops should be placed back on bottles to prevent spillages and a thorough skin analysis should be completed, to make sure there are no skin allergies to the product
Toner		Skin product that tightens the skin and removes excess traces of cleansing products	Tops should be placed back on bottles to prevent spillages and a thorough skin analysis should be completed, to make sure there are no skin allergies to the product
Moisturiser		A moisturising product helps to nourish dry areas of the skin, this gives a good base to apply make-up	Tops should be placed back on bottles to prevent spillages and a thorough skin analysis should be completed, to make sure there are no skin allergies to the product
Make-up palette		This tool is to prevent cross infection. It is designed to display the colours of the product you are about to use. You work from the palette and not the pots of make-up	By scraping small amounts of product on to the palette and working just from there, you are not going to contaminate the products by re-dipping into pots of make-up. Always make sure the palette is cleaned before and after treatments using a sanitising solution
Foundation		A product designed to even out skin tone and disguise minor blemishes	Always secure the lid tightly after use to avoid the product spoiling and accidental spillages. Make sure the client has no known allergies
Powder		A product designed to set the foundation, disguise minor blemishes and make the skin appear smooth and oil free	Always check that the client has no known allergies to the product ingredients before treatment
Eye shadows		A product to add colour and definition to the eye area, it can complement the client's eye colour and enhance the shape of the eye	Always check that the client has no known allergies to the product ingredients before treatment
Eyebrow liners		These define and emphasise the eye area	Always check that the client has no known allergies to the product ingredients before treatment

Product		Use	Health and safety
Blusher		Adds warmth to the face and shows the cheek bones off	Always check that the client has no known allergies to the product ingredients before treatment
Lipliners		Help to stop 'bleeding' of a dark lipstick. They can add definition to the lips by outlining them	Always check that the client has no known allergies to the product ingredients before treatment
Lipsticks/lip gloss		Add colour to the lip area, these product can add moisture to the lips	Always check that the client has no known allergies to the product ingredients before treatment
Mascara		This product makes the eyelashes appear longer, darker and thicker	Always check that the client has no known allergies to the product ingredients before treatment

Preparing the client

Help the client into a comfortable and relaxed position for the treatment. If you and your client are not comfortable it can cause discomfort and lead to possible injury.

Client consultation

In preparation for the client's basic make-up they will need to be consulted about their treatment needs. The information gained from the client is confidential and must not be given to anyone else. We must complete a client **consultation sheet** on which we record the information we have discovered and also to record that we have checked if the client has any conditions that may prevent or restrict treatment. It is also important that we check, by asking, if our client has any known allergies.

We need to carry out a basic skin analysis to check for any conditions that are not treatable. Sometimes we need to adapt the treatment or even, in extreme situations, postpone the treatment. When you carry out your consultation, it is always best to check with your tutor. The conditions we need to look for are in the list below.

ACTIVITY 007–5

Make a list of all the things you need to get ready for a treatment from memory.

Make sure your tutor has checked your work. Tick when you have completed this activity.

ACTIVITY 007-6

Find out more about skin disorders.

How we should deal with someone who has them. What they look like.

Make sure your tutor has checked your work. Tick when you have completed this activity.

Conditions which may prevent or restrict basic make-up treatment

Surrounding cuts and abrasions

Q. What does it look like?

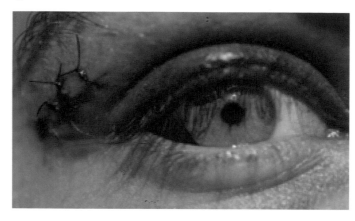

Q. Does it mean the treatment cannot go ahead?

A. If the cut or abrasion is open then you cannot treat the client due to the risk of cross infection.

Q. Does it mean the treatment can go ahead, but may need to be adapted?

A. If the cut or abrasion has healed then you can go ahead with the treatment but care should be taken when working over the area.

- *Always check with the tutor if you are unsure.*

Bruising and swelling

Q. What does it look like?

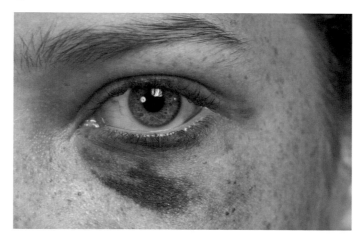

Q. Does it mean the treatment cannot go ahead?

A. The treatment can go ahead but you need to take care.

Q. Does it mean the treatment can go ahead, but may need to be adapted?

A. The treatment can be adapted by avoiding the area of bruising and swelling.

- *Always check with the tutor if you are unsure.*

Skin disorders

What does it look like?

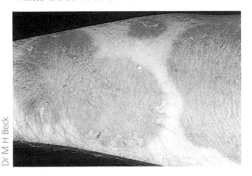

Psoriasis

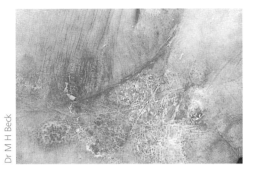

Eczema

Q. What are they called?

A. **Dermatitis, Eczema, Psoriasis**

● *Always check with the tutor if you are unsure.*

The treatment

1   Complete the record card/treatment plan, listing all the details of the treatment.

2   Wash your hands.

3   Ask your client to remove jewellery such as necklaces before you begin the treatment. This is recommended so skincare products do not soil the jewellery.

4   Place a head band on your client to avoid products getting into the hair.

5   A towel or a gown should be placed around the client to prevent products being spilt on to the client's clothes.

6   Complete a visual check of your client's skin, a skin analysis will identify skin types and conditions.

7   Gently remove any existing make-up from the clients skin, by following this routine:

● Each eye should be cleansed using a suitable eye make-up remover, support the skin as you sweep down the lashes with damp cotton wool pads soaked in the product.

● Apply cleanser to a damp cotton wool pad and sweep across the lips to remove any dirt, grime or old lip products.

● Apply cleanser to the client's skin using both your hands. Using sweeping effleurage movements working in upwards stokes.

● Remove the cleansing products in an upward and outward sweeping motion using damp cotton wool pads.

● Repeat this process, this time apply a suitable toner to damp cotton wool pads.

● Blot the skin dry with tissue.

● Apply a suitable moisturiser, use light sweeping movements.

KEY FACT

We sometimes need to adapt the treatment if the client has any of these conditions and in some cases we cannot go ahead. You may need to ask your tutor for help to explain this to the client.

REMEMBER

When completing a cleansing routine, select the correct range of products to suit your client's skin type. For example cleansers for a dry skin.

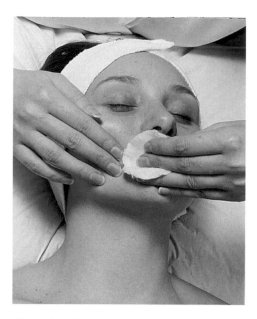

Cleansing the eye area

Cleansing the lips

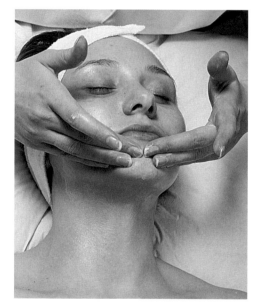

Cleansing the face

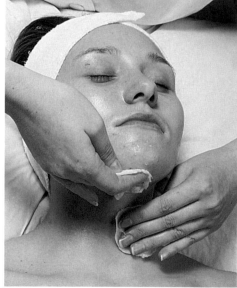

Removing cleanser

KEY FACT

Communication is important with your client; you must talk to your client throughout the treatment to make sure they know what you are doing. You need to discuss the colours they would like.

ACTIVITY 007–7

Find out more about the different types of cleansing products. How we should use them. Make a chart to list the products and state the skin types they are suitable for.

Make sure your tutor has checked your work. Tick when you have completed this activity.

ACTIVITY 007–8

Find out the different occasions on which a client might choose to have a make-up treatment and how this might affect the choice of products or colours.

Make sure your tutor has checked your work. Tick when you have completed this activity.

8 Once the skin has been prepared for a basic make-up treatment, the sequence in which you apply it is important. One reason is to avoid smudging the make-up.

9 Confirm with the client the occasion for the make-up treatment and check the type of colours they like. You may need to agree this at this stage.

10 Apply make-up in the following sequence:
- Foundation
- Powder
- Eye shadow

- Mascara
- Blusher
- Lipstick

11 Check with the client that the make-up has met their requirements.

12 Complete the treatment **record card**.

The purpose of a cleansing routine is to:

- Cleanse the skin to remove dirt and grime.
- Tone the skin to remove any remaining cleansing products.
- Moisturise the skin.
- Improve the blood circulation.
- Help to remove dead skin cells and improve the appearance of the skin.
- Prepare the client for a basic make-up treatment.

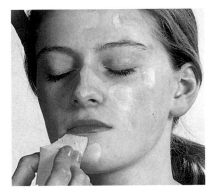

Applying foundation

Application techniques

Foundation

Apply the foundation over the entire face including the eyes and lips, this give an even cover, used a damp make-up sponge to get a nice even texture. Try to match the colour of the foundation to the client's skin colour, sometimes you need to mix two colours to get the right match, you can use your palette to do this.

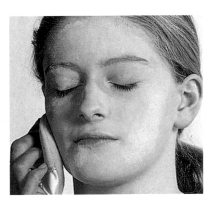

Applying powder

Powder

Face powder is applied to set the foundation, it can absorb oil from the skin so can take away the shine a skin can produce. A loose powder can be applied to the face with a big powder brush or soft sponge. Light soft strokes up and down the face makes sure the foundation is set.

Eye shadow

Eye shadows are available in powder or cream format. Either should be applied with an eye shadow brush or sponge applicator, never fingers, which could spread infections. You may need to experiment with different colours to get the effect you want. Eyeliners can come in pencil or liquid format, you need a steady hand to use liquid and it might be a good idea to practise on yourself first. Eyebrow pencils can be used to outline the eyebrow; make sure you use only light feathery movements. You must sharpen the pencil before and after use to prevent cross-infection.

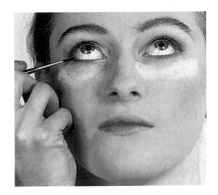

Applying eyeshadow

Mascara

A disposable mascara wand should always be used to reduce the risk of cross-infection. Applying mascara to a client can be difficult. Hold the brush horizontally and apply the colour to the length of the lashes, ask the client to look straight ahead.

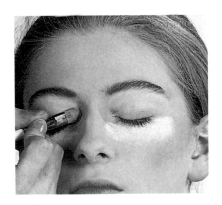

Applying eyeliner to the base lashline

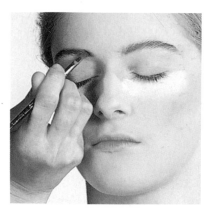

Applying eyebrow colour

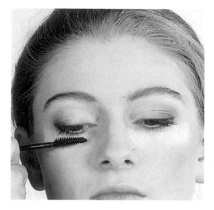

Applying mascara

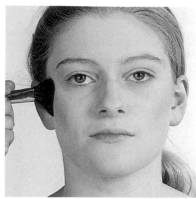

Applying blusher

Blusher

Applying blusher to the cheek area can change the appearance of the shape of the face. Remember it is easier to add more blusher than to take it away, so always apply a light application first and build up if needed. Sometimes the blusher or shading products can be applied to different areas of the face to alter the shape.

Face shapes: the four main face shapes and how blusher should be applied

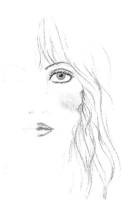

Oval

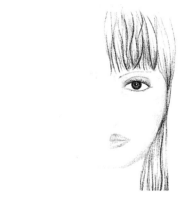

Round

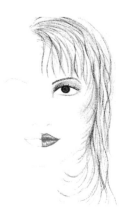

Square

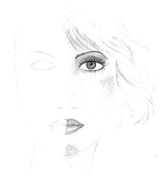

Oblong

Oval: thought of as the perfect face shape, apply the blusher to just underneath the cheek bones.

Round: apply blusher in a triangle shape with the base of the triangle running in front of the ear.

Square: apply blusher in a circular pattern on the cheek bone.

Oblong: apply blusher along the cheek bone outwards towards the ear.

Lipsticks, lip gloss and lipliners

Lip products come in lots of different formats. When choosing a lip product think about: the client's lips, skin and hair colour and if the product will suit the client. Use a lipliner to line the lips. Make sure you sharpen the pencil before and after use to prevent cross-infection. Then fill in the lips using a lipstick or lip gloss. It is important to scrape the lip stick on to the palette and not dip the lip brush or applicator into the product repeatedly to avoid cross-infection.

Completing the basic make-up treatment

Once we have finished the treatment there are some important things to remember.

- The client must like what we have achieved, so it is very important to check with them that they are satisfied.
- It is important we check for any reactions that may cause problems for the client, theses reactions are called **contra actions**.
- We need to give the client **aftercare** advice.
- We must update the record card.

Contra actions

Contra actions are reactions that can happen during or after the treatment and can develop up to 24 hours after the treatment. It is important that you look out for these reactions during treatment and advise your client to do the same once you have finished the treatment. These reactions are rare but can happen. The signs to look for are:

- Excessive perspiration.
- Watery eyes.
- Skin reactions/redness/swelling.

If any of the above happens, you must *stop* the treatment and *remove* the products *immediately*.

- Blot skin.
- Apply a soothing product.
- It is very important that you report this to your tutor. This is why it is so important to check for any known allergies during consultation prior to treatment. If you know your client has product allergies you can check to see if those ingredients are in the products you are going to use. If you

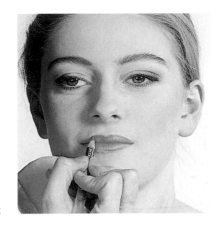

Applying lipliner

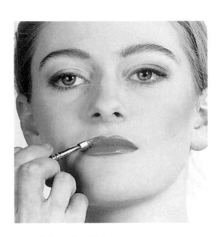

Applying lipstick

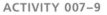

ACTIVITY 007–9

Find out what the different contra actions look like.

Make sure your tutor has checked your work. Tick when you have completed this activity.

are unsure check these with your tutor. Any reactions should be recorded on to the client's record card. The client may be recommended to seek medical advice.

Aftercare

The aftercare advice you give to a client is an important part of the treatment. This will differ from client to client, depending on their individual needs. The basic aftercare advice should include:

- Not to rub their eyes or to keep touching the face, as this could smudge the make-up.
- Apply the lipstick as needed.
- Always remove the make-up before going to sleep.
- Cleanse, tone and moisturise the skin with suitable products to match the client's skin type.

REMEMBER	✔

Always complete a treatment plan for every client you do and keep them in your portfolio.

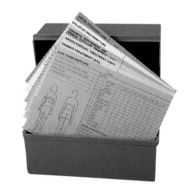

Ellisons

Record cards

Consultation sheet/record cards

It is very important to keep records of what treatments the client has received and what products you have used on them. You will need to state what colours and products you have used. If the client decides to return to have the treatment again and would like the same colours, you have a record of them. This means that you can repeat the successful processes at a later date with confidence. You could never remember all that information if it was not written down.

Some salons will keep client record cards, which record basic information, others will keep client consultation sheets, which record all that was done on every visit. Many salons now keep this information on their salon computer system. One advantage of this is that all sorts of reports can be generated to help the salon.

You should complete a client consultation sheet with all the details of what you have done on each client. It will help you develop your skills. To improve your skills you need to practise.

Key facts for you to remember from this chapter

- Keeping the salon clean will reduce the risk of transferring infections and diseases. It will also give the right impression to the client.

- Always complete a treatment plan and consultation for every client.

- Communication is important.

- Always give correct aftercare advice.

- Check for any conditions which may restrict or prevent the treatment.

- Check the product you are going to use suits the client's requirements.

- Complete a cleansing routine in the correct order.

- Apply make-up in the correct sequence.

- Have all tools and equipment near by when carrying out a treatment.

GLOSSARY

Aftercare   Information we give to a client at the end of a treatment to advise them on how to improve the condition of their skin or prolong the effect of the treatment.

Consultation sheet/record cards   Information sheet to record client details and treatment outcomes.

Contra actions   A reaction that can happen during or up to 24 hours after a treatment.

Dermatitis   An inflammatory skin disorder, in which the skin becomes dry, red and itchy.

Dermis   The inner portion of the skin, situated underneath the epidermis.

Eczema   Inflammation of the skin caused by contact internally or externally with an irritant.

Epidermis   Top layer of the skin.

Psoriasis   Patches of itchy red flaky skin.

Sanitation   prevents the multiplication of micro-organisms, but it does not kill all micro-organisms.

These are multiple-choice questions. Read the question carefully and then read the four possible answers. When you have decided which of the possible answers is the right one underline either a, b, c, or d in the box under the question.

1 Which of the following is present on a dry skin?
   a Large pores
   b Oily shine
   c Flaky skin
   d Blackheads

a	b	c	d

2 The function of a cleanser is to
   a Remove dirt and grime
   b Add colour to the skin
   c Moisturise the skin
   d Disguise impurities

a	b	c	d

3 What does mascara do?
   a Helps the lashes grow
   b Thicken the lashes
   c Curls the lashes
   d Evens out skin colour

a	b	c	d

4 In what order is the skin cleansed?
   a Cleanse, tone and moisturise
   b Moisturise, tone and cleanse
   c Tone, cleanse and moisturise
   d Cleanse, moisturise and tone

a	b	c	d

Questions to test your knowlege of this unit (cont.)

Now try the following short answer questions. These may need a single word to answer or a short sentence or list.

1 Name three tools that would be used in a make-up treatment and state what each does.

Answer   1. _____

2. _____

3. _____

2 Why do we complete a treatment plan on a client?

Answer _____

_____

3 State the four face shapes.

Answer   1. _____

2. _____

3. _____

4. _____

4 List three things that you should remember when you are giving aftercare advice.

Answer   1. _____

2. _____

3. _____

Helpful hints for the assignment

Introduction to the assignment

The assignment looks at what you have been learning about in this chapter: trends in make-up products, designs and techniques.

Your tutor will give you the assignment and guide you on the maximum time you should allow to be sure of completing all of the course assignments.

Where to look for examples

You will need to find examples of products, designs and techniques used. You can find this type of information on the Internet, trade magazines, fashion magazines and advertising material. You may also use photographs of clients you have treated, showing the end results of your practical work to demonstrate products and techniques. However your assignment needs to be in your own words.

Presentation decisions

Remember to give a description of the pictures or images you have selected. What is your opinion of these? You can use a computer to type these comments or neatly hand write them. When sticking in pictures think about how it will look. You may decide to cut and paste pictures or images.

Structure

You should start with an introduction, explaining what you are going to do, and say what you are going to find out. Complete your report with some conclusions.

Remember to include references (where your information came from).

Don't forget that presentation is important for this task.

CHECKERBOARD

After you have completed the chapter on Applying Basic Make-up, rate yourself on the checkerboard. (You must be honest with yourself, don't put a tick in the box if you haven't done the work or don't feel that you have learned what you need to know.)

I can set up the work area on my own □	I can carry out a consultation □	I can use positive body language □	I know a basic make-up treatment □
I know what all the products are used for □	I know the sequence of the treatment □	I know why teamwork is important in the salon □	I am aware of the health and safety needed when completing a treatment □
I know the basic structure of the skin □	I know the conditions which restrict and prevent treatment □	I know the basic skin types □	I can use the make-up products in the correct sequence □
I can give a client the correct aftercare advice □	I can tidy my work area without being reminded □	I can name the functions of the skin □	I know what to do if a reaction happens □

CHECKER BOARD ✓

ACTIVITY CHECKLIST

Make sure you have completed all the activities linked to this chapter and that you have put any information you need to keep in your portfolio.

Only tick the box and complete the portfolio reference when your tutor has confirmed the activity is complete.

	Complete	Portfolio Reference
Activity 007–1 (p. 114)	☐	
Activity 007–2 (p. 114)	☐	
Activity 007–3 (p. 115)	☐	
Activity 007–4 (p. 116)	☐	
Activity 007–5 (p. 119)	☐	
Activity 007–6 (p. 120)	☐	
Activity 007–7 (p. 122)	☐	
Activity 007–8 (p. 122)	☐	
Activity 007–9 (p. 125)	☐	

chapter 8

UNIT 008 PROVIDING BASIC MANICURE

Introduction

In this chapter we are going to cover the skills and knowledge you will need to prepare the client, set up the working area and carry out a basic manicure.

The main assessment requirement for this unit will be practical observations, where you will carry out the practical tasks we are going to look at in this chapter. There is also an assignment that you will complete. As a result of your practical work and the work we will do in this chapter, which will support your practical work, you will need to show that you are able to:

- **Prepare your work area.**
- **Prepare your client for the treatment.**
- **Carry out a consultation and complete a treatment plan.**
- **Carry out a basic manicure treatment.**
- **Recognise nail shapes.**
- **Identify the basic nail structure.**
- **List the conditions which may prevent or restrict treatments.**
- **Outline reactions which may occur and how you would deal with them.**
- **Understand how to use the products and equipment needed to carry out a manicure.**
- **Carry out a basic nail art treatment.**

When we carry out a basic manicure, it is important at all times to follow all the things we learnt in Chapter 4 Following Health and Safety Practice and Chapter 1 Finding out about Customer Service.

Remember your practical observations will be carried out by your tutor and, if you have completed the requirements of the observation criteria, they will sign off the task. For the tasks in this unit you will be observed several times before your tutor will finally sign off all tasks. You can gain a pass, credit or distinction in this element. Your tutor will explain what this means during your induction.

WHAT YOU NEED TO KNOW

To complete the assignment which is part of the assessment for this unit you will need to:

● Find out the current and emerging trends within the nail industry.

● Produce a nail care book to show examples of nail products, designs, techniques and trends

During the practical observation you will need to demonstrate that you can:

● Prepare your work area ready for your client.

● Have all your equipment ready to use.

● Carry out a consultation and complete a treatment plan.

● Carry out a basic manicure treatment.

● Discuss the aftercare advice with your client.

● Clean your work area.

Remember the quality of your completed assignment can gain you a pass, credit or distinction.

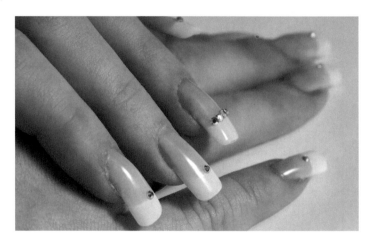

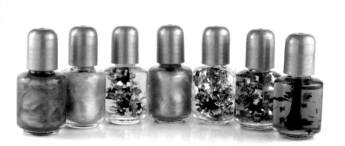

A MANICURE

The basic manicure treatment aims to improve the appearance of:

● Hands

● Cuticles

● Nails.

Hands

Healthy hands have soft, smooth skin. Wear and tear, or neglect, can make the skin dry, chapped, sore and rough.

When we carry out a basic manicure, our aim is to maintain the soft, smooth skin or return the skin to a healthy, soft, smooth condition. This might take more than one treatment. We will need to advise our client on how they can look after their hands and nails at home. This is called aftercare advice.

Cuticles

The cuticle is the part of the skin found around the base of the nail. When it's healthy and in good condition it is soft and loose. When it is not being looked after it can become dry, tight and overgrown and can split, which can become sore.

Nails

The nail should be smooth, supple and have a healthy pink appearance. The edge that is filed should be even, this is called the free edge. Nails can lose their healthy pink colour and can become ridged, brittle and flaky if they are not looked after. The surface of the nail is called the nail plate. When we carry out a basic manicure treatment our aim is to maintain or improve the healthy pink colour of the nail.

> **KEY FACT** !
>
> Nails grow faster in the summer than winter.
>
> Faster in young people than in older.
>
> Faster on the hand you use most.
>
> Illness or medication can affect nail growth, either speeding it up or slowing it down.

ANATOMY AND PHYSIOLOGY

As we discovered in Chapter 7, we must learn about the structure of the body and how it works. For this chapter we need to learn about the nails, their structure, how they grow and their functions.

The basic nail unit

Nails grow from the ends of the fingers and toes and their main purpose is to form a hard protective shield.

The nail plate

The nail plate is the correct name for the part of the nail that covers the nail bed, the portion of the skin on which the nail plate rests. The cells here are clear and have become hardened. These hard cells are there to protect the nail bed below and, because they are clear, allow you to see if the living nail bed is a healthy pink colour. The function of the nail plate is to protect the nail bed. The nail grows forward slowly over the nail bed at the rate of 0.5mm to 1.2mm per week. It takes between 4 and 6 months for a nail plate to grow fully from the cuticle to free edge.

The nail bed

The nail bed is the part of the skin covered by the nail plate. The nail plate and the nail bed separate at the free edge (end of the finger). The nail bed is made up of living cells and contains blood vessels, which help to keep it healthy and allow for the nail to grow and repair itself. The nail bed also contains nerves which enable you to feel pain, heat etc.

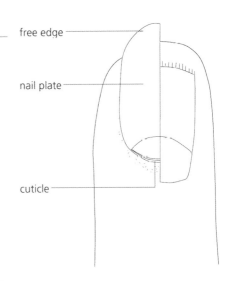

free edge —

nail plate —

cuticle —

The structure of the nail

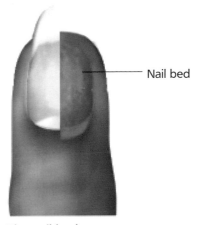

— Nail bed

The nail bed

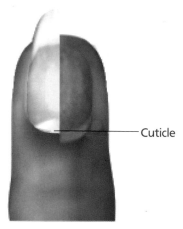

— Cuticle

The cuticle

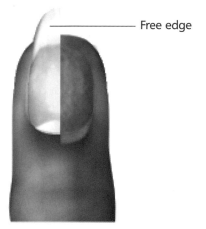

——————— Free edge

The free edge

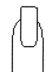 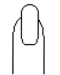

Oval, Square, Fan

KEY FACT !

Keeping the salon clean will reduce the risk of transferring infections and diseases. It will also give the right impression to the client.

REMEMBER ✔

If you do not have anything to do then clean and tidy anything that needs it. Teamwork and helping colleagues is important.

The cuticle

The cuticle is the overlapping skin at the bottom of the nail plate that grows forward on to the nail plate. When the cuticle becomes dry it can often split and possibly become infected. It is important to keep the cuticles soft and loose. The function of the cuticle is to protect the nail plate.

The free edge

The free edge is the part of the nail that grows beyond the finger tip. It is usually white, as it does not lie on top of the pink nail bed. This is the part of the nail that you can file and shape. The function of the free edge is to protect the finger nail.

NAIL SHAPES

Each client's hands, fingers and nails are different. It is important that the nail shape and length suits their hands. The free edge can be shaped to improve the appearance of the hands and fingers. The types of nail shapes are:

- Oval: the sides of the free edge are curved. This is an ideal shape for short, stubby fingers as it makes the fingers appear slimmer and longer.
- Square: the free edge is filed straight across. This nail shape will improve the appearance of long thin fingers.
- Squoval: a combination of oval and square nail shapes. The nail is filed to a square finish at the free edge and then gently curved at the corners.

CARRYING OUT A BASIC MANICURE

Preparing the work area

There are lots of things we need to consider in the preparation of our working area and for the treatment itself. Whether we use a table, manicure station or work surface we need to think about the health and safety precautions involved:

- Is the floor area clean and free from spillages or anything else?
- Is the chair and work surface clean?
- If there is a trolley is it clean and tidy?
- Is the equipment to hand?

Remember our work on impressions in Chapters 1 and 2, make sure the client gets the right impression when they are brought to the salon or work area. A clean work area shows you take care and pride in your work.

Carrying out a basic manicure treatment involves sanitising the work area and using tools and products which can be disposed of or cleaned quite easily.

The work area must be wiped over with a sanitising solution before and after treatment.

- Place a clean towel over the work area.
- Fold another towel into a pad and place it in the middle of the work surface (this will help to support the client's forearm).
- You will need a further small towel to dry your client's hands during the treatment.
- A piece of couch roll or tissue should be placed on top of the towels.
- A lined bin should be placed beside the working area
- Position a stool or chair for yourself and the client.

There are some other points to consider when setting up and selecting our tools, equipment and products. The chart below includes the products, tools and equipment you may use, as well as health and safety factors that need to be followed.

> **REMEMBER**
>
> Dispose of all waste products in a lined bin.

Product	Use	Health and safety
Sanitising solution Ellisons	To wipe over treatment work area and surface. Sanitising liquid prevents the multiplication of micro-organisms, but it does not kill all micro-organisms	Could cause a slippage if spilt. Might cause skin irritation and could be toxic if swallowed. Chemical sterilising sprays are also used to sanitise the surface of the work area. These should be used following manufacturer's instructions and in a well ventilated area. Avoid contact with flame and excessive heat
Finger bowl	Fill with warm water and add a pleasant smelling nail soak to cleanse and soften the cuticles	Clean before and after use with a detergent, disinfectant and sanitising solution. Rinse well and dry thoroughly. When in use keep on a stable surface to avoid spillage
Emery board Ellisons	A nail file that is used to shape the nails. It usually has two sides, one side is coarser than the other	Use a different emery board for each client to avoid cross-infection. The coarse side is used to reduce the length of the nail. Never use a sawing action when filing as you can cause the free edge to split
Orange sticks Ellisons	Disposable wooden tools, usually with a hoof shaped end for use around the cuticle and a pointed end for cleaning under the free edge. They can also be used to remove product from containers.	Never reuse the orange stick, throw away after each treatment to avoid cross-infection. Always tip with clean cotton wool if using under the free edge. If used incorrectly they could damage the nail or surrounding skin
Cuticle cream	To restore oil to the surrounding skin of the nail and to the nail plate itself	Cuticle creams are added in small quantities to the nail and surrounding skin. It is important not to dip fingers into the pot, always use an orange stick taking care not to re-dip it (**cut out method**)

Product	Use	Health & Safety
Nail polish remover Ellisons	A product that will dissolve and remove nail polish and any grease from the nail plate. The active ingredient that causes this to happen is acetone	Nail polish remover can be drying to the nail and the surrounding skin, choose one that contains moisturising oils. Store away from heat as it is highly flammable
Base coat Salon System	It is essential that base coat is used before applying a nail polish. It gives the nail added protection and prevents a coloured polish from staining the nail plate.	Always secure the lid tightly after use to avoid the product spoiling and accidental spillages. Make sure the client has no known allergies to nail polishes
Nail polish Salon System	Can be applied to improve the natural appearance of the nail, or add colour and protection	Always secure the lid tightly after use to avoid the product spoiling and accidental spillages. Make sure the client has no known allergies to nail polishes
Top coat Salon System	This is applied only on top of a cream nail polish. It gives sheen to the nail. Pearlised polishes do not need a top coat. It provides a colourless protective film to the nail polish.	Always secure the lid tightly after use to avoid the product spoiling and accidental spillages. Make sure the client has no known allergies to nail polishes
Nail strengtheners Salon System	A product designed to help with fragile or brittle nails. It can contain formaldehyde	Always secure the lid tightly after use to avoid the product spoiling and accidental spillages. Make sure the client has no known allergies to **formaldehyde**
Hand soak	A product that can be added to the warm water, to cleanse and soften the cuticles	Always check that the client has no known allergies to the product ingredients before treatment
Hand cream Salon System	A product designed to moisturise the skin and nails. It provides the slip when massaging the area	Some hand creams contain **lanolin** which may cause an allergic reaction. Always check with the client before use

Preparing the client

Help the client into a comfortable and relaxed position for the treatment. If you and your client are not comfortable it can cause discomfort and lead to possible injury.

Client consultation

In preparation for the client's basic manicure treatment, we will need to consult with them about their treatment needs. The information we gain from the client is confidential and must not be given to anyone else. We must complete a client consultation sheet on which we record the information we have discovered and also to record that we have checked if the client has any conditions that may prevent or restrict treatment. It is also important that we check, by asking, if our client has any known allergies.

The next stage is to inspect your client's hands and nails, if you see anything you are unsure of it is always best to check with your tutor before continuing. The types of conditions we are looking for are:

- Cuts or abrasions surrounding the nails or on the hands.
- Bruising or swelling of the hands and fingers.
- Severe nail damage.

Sometimes treatments need to be adapted or, in extreme situations, postponed. You may need to ask for help to explain this to your client.

The treatment

1 Complete the record card/treatment plan, listing all the details of the treatment.

2 Wash your hands.

3 Ask the client to remove all jewellery before you begin the treatment. This is recommended so massage creams do not soil the jewellery.

4 Complete a visual check of the client's hands and nails.

5 If the client is wearing nail polish this must be removed so we can see our client's nail condition. Use the following procedure:

- Soak a clean piece of cotton wool in nail polish remover, place this on to the clients nail plate and wait for 2–3 seconds. The nail polish should start to dissolve.
- Apply firm downward strokes from the cuticle to the free edge.
- Any remaining polish left around the cuticle area can be removed using a tipped orange stick soaked in nail polish remover.
- Look at the nails closely to see if any are dry, flaky chipped or peeling, this could show the nails are dry or dehydrated.
- Are the nails discoloured?
- What shape are the client's nails and what shape would they like?
- Are the nails bitten?

6 Assess the condition of the client's skin on their hands and arms. Things to look for:

- Are the cuticles dry, tight or split, or are they soft and supple?
- Is the skin on the hands and arms dry, flaky, tight or rough, or smooth and soft.

7 Using the fine side of an emery board shape the natural free edge. Confirm with the client the nail shape and length during this stage and make any alterations. Use the dark or rougher side of the emery board to reduce length.

8 Check all nails are even and have smooth edges, check with the client.

9 Massage cuticle cream into the cuticles of all nails on the hand.

10 Place hand in finger bowl containing hand soak and repeat the filing and cuticle cream steps on the other hand.

11 Dry the first hand thoroughly and gently roll back cuticles with tipped orange stick. Gently push back cuticles taking care not to push too hard. Repeat this step on the second hand.

12 Apply massage cream to the first hand and arm and complete a massage sequence, repeat on the second hand.

- Effleurage from fingers to elbow × 3 each side.
- Thumb frictions to the wrist.
- Thumb frictions to the back of the hand × 3.
- Thumb frictions to the fingers.
- Circle the fingers slowly each way one at a time × 3.
- Wrist circles × 3.
- Thumb circles to the palm of the hand × 3.
- Petrissage to the forearm working from wrist to elbow × 3.
- Effleurage to the elbow × 3.
- Effleurage from the finger to the elbow × 3.

13 Remove any cream from the free edge using a tipped orange stick.

14 Squeak the nails with nail polish remover, making sure there are no traces of oil or cream left.

15 Check the nail shape and length with the client. Bevel the tips if necessary to make sure the free edge is smooth.

16 Apply base coat.

17 Apply two coats of nail polish.

18 Apply a top coat if using a cream polish.

The purpose of massage is to:

- Moisturise the skin.
- Improve the blood circulation.
- Help to remove dead skin cells and improve the appearance of the skin.
- Relax the client.

The three types of massage movements we use in hand and arm massage are:

Effleurage – this is a soft stroking movement that we use to spread the massage cream or oil. It always begins and finishes any massage routine.

Petrissage – this is a deeper kneading movement that helps to increase circulation and ease tense and tight muscles.

Friction – this is a small circular movement performed with either fingers or thumbs. It can be a deep movement pressure.

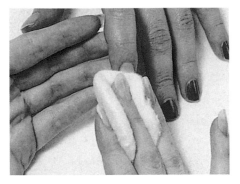

Removing nail polish

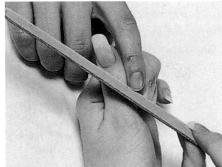

Filing

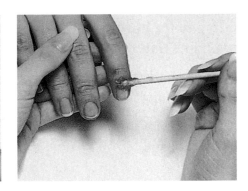

Applying cuticle cream

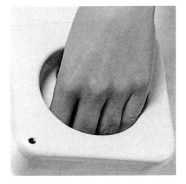

One hand in a bowl

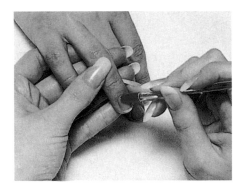

Pushing back cuticles

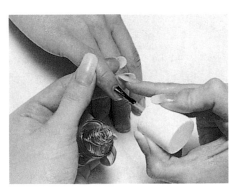

Applying the base coat

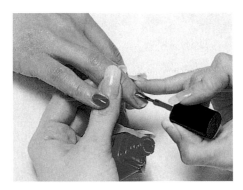

Applying nail polish

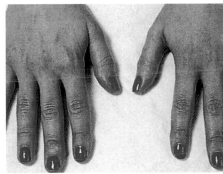

The completed manicure

Nail painting techniques

Nail polish is applied to the nail plate for the following reasons:

- To improve the appearance of the client's hands and nails.
- To add strength to nails.
- To disguise stained nails.
- For a special occasion.

1   Select the nail polish agreed with your client.
2   Apply the base coat, nail polish and top coat, if applicable, in this order.

REMEMBER

It is important to practise your nail painting to avoid flooding the cuticles with nail colour. Take your time. Having too much polish on the brush will cause flooding. Make sure your bottle tops are cleaned after use as this will help the product to stay in good condition.

3 Unscrew the bottle top to which a brush is attached. Wipe the brush on one side against the neck of the bottle, turn the brush around and apply the side of the brush with the polish to the nail.

4 Starting with the thumb apply three strokes down the nail plate starting at the cuticle; avoid contact to the cuticle with the polish. The first stroke is usually down the centre then one on each side.

5 Apply just one coat of base coat.

6 Apply the nail polish in the same way.

7 Apply two coats of nail polish.

8 Apply a top coat.

Nail Art

Nail art is the technique of creating artistic designs on the nail using a range of decorative materials.

If you are going to use nail art on your client it comes at the end of the manicure. It is always nice to complete a manicure first so the nails and surrounding skin are in good condition. Some of the techniques involved are as follows.

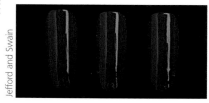

Jefford and Swain

Japanese symbol

This is a free hand technique using a fine brush. First your client chooses the block colour for the nail plate and then the symbol can be applied using light pressure to apply fine lines and heavier pressure to apply thicker lines.

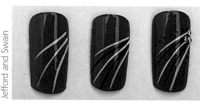

Jefford and Swain

Striping design

Different brushes are used to make stripes of colour. You can purchase self-adhesive strips to apply to the nail plate to create this effect.

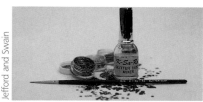

Jefford and Swain

Glitter dust

This is a fine sparkly powder available in different colours which are applied with a brush. A sealer needs to be applied to seal the design.

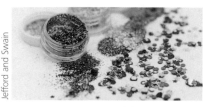

Jefford and Swain

Flat stones and rhinestone

Tiny stones or gems available in different sizes and colours are secured to the nail polish whilst it is still wet.

Jefford and Swain

Transfers

These are images that can be secured to the nail creating an instant design.

Nail art is lots of fun. You can develop your own designs. All you need are the simple tools, products and lots of time.

Completing the nail treatment

Once we have finished the treatment there are some important things to remember.

- The client must like what we have achieved, so it is very important to check with them that they are satisfied.
- It is important we check for any reactions that may cause problems for the client. These reactions are called **contra actions**.
- We need to give the client aftercare advice.
- We must update the record card.

Contra actions

Contra actions are reactions that can happen during or after the treatment and can develop up to 24 hours after the treatment. It is important that we look out for these reactions during treatment and advise our client to do the same once we have finished the treatment. These reactions are rare but can happen. The signs to look for are:

- Redness
- Irritation
- Swelling

If any of the above happens, we must **stop** the treatment and **remove** the products **immediately**. It is very important that you report this to your tutor. This is why it is so important that we ask the client about allergies and sensitivity and that we look at the skin and nails during the consultation stage. If we know our client has product allergies we should check to see if those ingredients are in the products we are going to use. If you are unsure check these with your tutor. Any reactions should be recorded on to the **client's consultation sheet/record card**.

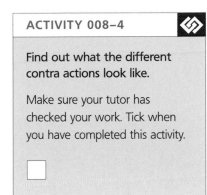

ACTIVITY 008–4

Find out what the different contra actions look like.

Make sure your tutor has checked your work. Tick when you have completed this activity.

Aftercare

The **aftercare** advice we give to a client is an important part of the treatment. This will differ from client to client, depending on their individual needs. The basic aftercare advice should include:

- Wear rubber gloves for washing up.
- Wear protective gloves when gardening.
- Dry the hands thoroughly after washing.
- Apply hand cream regularly, to moisturise the skin.
- Avoid harsh, drying soaps.
- Do not use the fingernails as tools, this causes the nails to weaken.
- Advise the client to have regular manicure treatments (on a monthly basis).

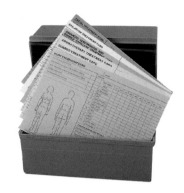

Record cards

REMEMBER ✔

Always complete a treatment plan for every client you do and keep them in your portfolio.

Consultation sheet/record cards

It is very important to keep records of what treatments our client has. It makes sure we can continue to keep out client's nails and hands in the best condition. It also provides information about the treatments and services we have carried out on the client. Things like the products that were used, how they were used and, most importantly, the results. This means that we can repeat the successful processes at a later date with confidence. We could never remember all that information in our head.

Some salons will keep client record cards which record basic information, others will keep client consultation sheets which record all that was done on every visit. Many salons now keep this information on their salon computer system. One advantage of this is that all sorts of reports can be generated to help the salon.

We should complete a client consultation sheet with all the details of what we have done on each of our clients. It will help us develop our skills. To improve our skills we need to practice.

Key facts for you to remember from this chapter

- Keeping the salon clean will reduce the risk of transferring infections and diseases. It will also give the right impression to the client.

- Always complete a treatment plan and consultation for every client.

- Communication is important.

- Always give correct aftercare advice.

- Check for any conditions which may restrict or prevent the treatment.

- It is important to practise your nail painting.

- The massage movements used in hand and arm massage are:

  Effleurage

  Petrissage

  Friction

- Never file down the sides of the nails.

- Have all tools and equipment near by when carrying out a treatment.

GLOSSARY

Aftercare   Information we give to a client at the end of a treatment to advise them on how to improve the condition or prolong the effect of the treatment.

Consultation sheet/record cards   Information sheet to record client details and treatment outcomes.

Contra actions   A reaction that can happen during or up to 24 hours after a treatment.

Cut out method   A procedure used to prevent cross-infection, by using a disposable tool to decant products without having to use your fingers or re-dip into containers.

Effleurage   Soft stroking massage movement.

Formaldehyde   An ingredient used in some nail products that can cause severe reactions.

Friction   Small circular massage movement which can be performed with fingers or thumbs.

Lanolin   An ingredient that comes from sheep's wool and can cause allergic reactions.

Nail art   A technique used to produce patterns on the nail.

Petrissage   Deeper kneading massage movement.

Questions to test your knowlege of this unit

These are multiple-choice questions. Read the question carefully and then read the four possible answers. When you have decided which of the possible answers is the right one underline either a, b, c, or d in the box under the question.

1 Which of the following is a soft stroking movement used in the hand and arm massage?

a Effleurage

b Petrissage

c Friction

d Rotary

a	b	c	d

2 The function of a base coat is to

a Protect the nails

b Strengthen the nails

c Colour the nails

d Lengthen the nails

a	b	c	d

3 What does cuticle cream do?

a Remove nail polish from nails

b Moisturises the hands and arms

c Restores oil to nail plate and cuticle

d Helps the nails to grow strong

a	b	c	d

4 What colour is the free edge?

a Pink

b White

c Skin colour

d Red

a	b	c	d

Questions to test your knowlege of this unit (cont.)

Now try the following short answer questions. These may need a single word to answer or a short sentence or list.

1 Name three tools that would be used in a manicure treatment and state what each does.

Answer 1. _____

2. _____

3. _____

2 Why do we carry out a consultation on a client?

Answer _____

_____

3 State the three most common nail shapes.

Answer 1. _____

2. _____

3. _____

4 List three things that you should remember when you are giving aftercare advice.

Answer 1. _____

2. _____

3. _____

Helpful hints for the assignment

Introduction to the assignment

The assignment looks at what you have been learning about in this chapter: current trends in nail products, different nail designs and techniques and trends in nail treatments.

Your tutor will give you the assignment and guide you on the maximum time you should allow to be sure of completing all of the course assignments.

Where to look for examples

You will need to find examples of products, designs and techniques used. You can find this type of information on the Internet, in trade magazines, fashion magazines and advertising material. You may also use photographs of clients you have treated, showing the end results of your practical work to demonstrate products and techniques. However your assignment needs to be in your own words.

Presentation decisions

Remember to give a description of the pictures or images you have selected. What is your opinion of these? You can use a computer to type these comments or neatly hand write them. When sticking in pictures think about how it will look. You may decide to cut and paste pictures or images.

Structure

You should start with an introduction, explaining what you are going to do, and say what you are going to find out. Complete your report with some conclusions. Don't forget to include references (where your information came from).

Don't forget that presentation is important for this task.

CHECKERBOARD

After you have completed the chapter on Providing Basic Manicure, rate yourself on the checkerboard. (You must be honest with yourself, don't put a tick in the box if you haven't done the work or don't feel that you have learned what you need to know.)

I can set up the work area on my own ☐	I can carry out a consultation ☐	I can use positive body language ☐	I know the basic manicure routine ☐
I know what all the products are used for ☐	I know the sequence of the treatment ☐	I know why teamwork is important in the salon ☐	I am aware of the health and safety needed when completing a treatment ☐
I know the basic structure of the nail ☐	I know the conditions which restrict and prevent treatment ☐	I know the hand and arm massage routine ☐	I can paint the nails using the correct products ☐
I can give a client the correct aftercare advice ☐	I can tidy my work area without being reminded ☐	I can recognise nail shapes ☐	I know what to do if a reaction happens ☐

CHECKER BOARD ✓

ACTIVITY CHECKLIST

Make sure you have completed all the activities linked to this chapter and that you have put any information you need to keep in your portfolio.

Only tick the box and complete the portfolio reference when your tutor has confirmed the activity is complete.

	Complete	Portfolio Reference
Activity 008–1 (p. 139)	☐	
Activity 008–2 (p. 139)	☐	
Activity 008–3 (p. 140)	☐	
Activity 008–4 (p. 143)	☐	

chapter 9

UNIT 009 INDUSTRY AND OCCUPATIONAL AWARENESS

Introduction

So far we have learned about the skills we need to provide a high quality service to our clients.

In this chapter we will look at career development. Discover how you can plan your career. Find out the things you need to know about being employed. Find out where you can get advice and information to help you.

> For the assessment of this unit you will need to show that you:
>
> - **Understand the career structure of the hair and beauty industry.**
>
> - **Are aware of the career opportunities available in the industry.**
>
> - **Are aware of the types and levels of jobs in the industry.**
>
> - **Know how to access training for career progression and where to get information.**
>
> - **Are aware of your rights and your responsibilities as an employee in a salon.**

Your assessment for this unit is the completion of an assignment.

The assignment will be completed over a period of time and will involve researching information and then putting that information together in a report.

WHAT YOU NEED TO KNOW

To complete the assignment you have to do as part of the assessment for unit 009 you will need to:

- Find out about the organisations that provide information about working in hair and beauty salons.
- Find out about jobs available in the industry and the skills that are needed to do them.
- Find out about career development opportunities.
- Find out about your rights and responsibilities as an employee.

In addition you will need to be able to describe:

- The jobs available in a range of outlets.
- Career progression in the industry.
- What training and qualifications are available.
- The basic rights of an employee during their employment.

CAREER OPPORTUNITIES

There is a wide range of job opportunities available in the hair and beauty industry. The obvious ones are those in hairdressing and beauty salons, which we have concentrated on so far in our studies. There are lots of other opportunities for those who want more than just working in a salon.

- Hotels and cruise liners will have salon facilities to match their status (star rating) and will seek staff to match.
- **Health farms** and hydros will offer a wide range of jobs particularly to beauty therapists. They will be looking for specialists in all aspects of beauty therapy work. They will also have opportunities for hairdressers.
- Health and fitness clubs and leisure centres will have opportunities for specialist beauty therapists, for example those qualified in sports massage and other sport specific techniques.
- Hairdressers and specialists in make-up can find opportunities in the film, theatre and television field.
- Jobs in the fashion and photographic industry will appeal to those who want a career at the sharp end of fashion and innovation.
- The development of opportunities in the health service includes hairdressing services for patients and, increasingly, the use of some specialist beauty therapy techniques.
- We should not forget the retail industry, where a variety of opportunities exists in demonstrating and selling cosmetics and associated products.

If we are going to make the most of our decision to be a hairdresser or beauty therapist then we must find out about these opportunities.

REMEMBER

To progress your career you must know what opportunities are available to you and what you need (qualifications, experience etc.) to go for them.

ACTIVITY 009–1

Find out and write down the many jobs linked to hairdressing and beauty in the places listed below. Try and find out what qualifications you might need to apply for them.

- In a hotel
- On a cruise liner
- On a health farm or a hydro
- In a health and fitness club
- In the theatre, film and TV studios
- In the fashion and photography industry
- In hospitals
- In retail shops

Make sure your tutor has checked your work. Tick when you have completed this activity.

☐

HINT ★

Use trade magazines and the internet to help you find out. Look at the job vacancies section.

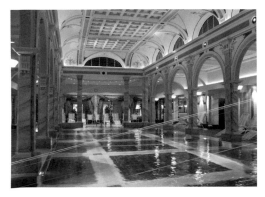 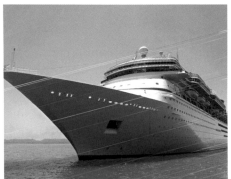 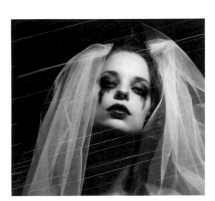

There are a range of career opportunities available to hairdressers and beauty therapists

PROGRESSING YOUR CAREER

The course you are now taking is your first step on the career ladder for a successful future as a hairdresser or beauty therapist. It is important to explore how we progress to the next step and then the next and also to find out what other directions are open to us.

Achieving the Salon Services Certificate will be useful to help you access your next move. How can you continue your development? You could take an 'apprenticeship' where you work and train in a salon, or work/train and study at college. You could also consider training on a full-time course at college.

We should start by looking at salon staffing structures.

The staff structure in a hairdressing salon will vary. The larger the salon the more complicated the structure could be, the smaller the salon the simpler the structure will be. This is normally influenced by the number of people who work there.

ACTIVITY 009–2

Make a brief plan of how you see your career developing in the next 3–4 years. Start with what you are doing now and include what you need to achieve to progress.

Make sure your tutor has checked your work. Tick when you have completed this activity.

☐

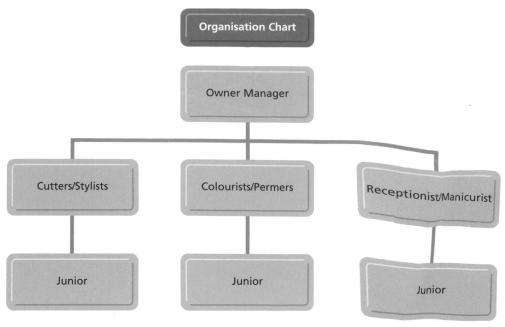

An example of an organisation chart for a hairdressing salon

At the bottom will be the 'junior' (which is what you would be at the start of your career, if you choose the 'apprenticeship' route). The junior assists the qualified staff and carries out some parts of the service the client has.

Next will be the hairdressers, sometimes they are called stylists or cutters. It will vary from salon to salon. Larger salons may have **colourists**, who carry out all the hair colouring in the salon, and other staff who specialise in different services. Above the hairdressers will be the manager or owner who will run the salon.

Some salons, especially large ones, have more rows in their chart with different titles for the staff.

In a beauty salon the structure may be different; the industry does not recruit as many juniors as hairdressers do. The majority of beauty therapists train through the 'college' route.

There is also a very wide range of specialisms that can be developed, manicurists and nail specialists, specialist massage techniques, **electrolysis**, and holistic therapies such as **reflexology**, **aromatherapy** etc.

The structure in the salon will, therefore, be mainly beauty therapists who provide a range of services for the client and then the specialists. Like hairdressing there will be a manager or owner running the salon.

These are just some examples to show you how you can progress in your career.

To make that progress you need to continue to learn. Skills and knowledge are essential for your career. In the beginning you must learn a wide range of skills and the knowledge and understanding that supports those skills. You will not be a professional hairdresser or beauty therapist if you have skills to provide services but do not understand what is happening or why. Not knowing what and why is very dangerous and could cause serious mistakes to be made and even serious injury to your client.

KEY FACT

To progress in your career you need qualifications including GCSEs, skills and knowledge.

Make sure you work hard to get the best qualifications you can.

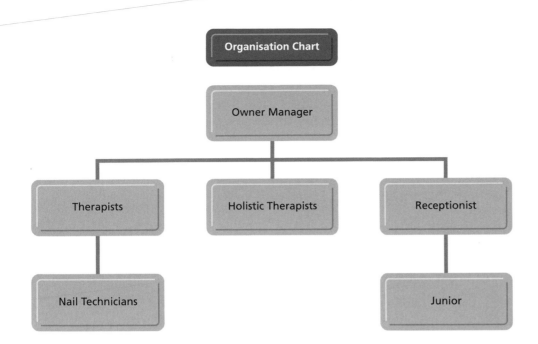

An example of an organisation chart for a beauty salon

When you have completed your 'apprenticeship' or training programme you can begin to move up the organisation chart. But don't forget, to do that you will need to have the qualifications, the skills and knowledge, the personal presentation, the customer service skills and the personality. All the things we have looked at in previous chapters.

At this point you should begin to think about your strengths, what you are good at or enjoy doing. This may persuade you to take another direction in your career. There may be opportunities for you to specialise earlier, for example to become a nail technician you can take a programme that does not contain all the other aspects of beauty therapy. There is a very wide range of opportunities open to you. Here are some examples:

- Make up artist or hairdresser in the film, TV, theatre or in the fashion industry.
- Specialist therapist in things like sports injury massage and other specific massage therapies.
- Aromatherapist, reflexologist, electrologist.
- Camouflage make-up for people with disfigurements.
- Sales representative or demonstrator for a cosmetic company.
- Wigmaker.
- Product development and research.
- **Trichologist**.
- Salon management.
- Teaching and training.

We have looked at what you can aspire to in your career if you work hard and get your qualifications and your skills. What we need to do now is to find out what qualifications you will need and other information about them that would be useful. We also need to find out how and where we can get support for career development.

There are many opportunities available to you either to start your training or to progress. The Connexions Service provides impartial advice and support to young people to help them find the information they need and help them to use it. Information from an awarding body (this is an organisation that provides the qualifications you might need to take) such as City & Guilds will tell you all about a qualification and where you can go to take it.

Other organisations like HABIA (this stands for the Hairdressing and Beauty Industry Authority) will provide information about the industry and the qualifications. They will say what has to be included in a qualification.

Your local college of further education or **training provider** will help you secure a route for progression, especially in the initial stages and also for a lot of specialist directions.

The range of qualifications that you can achieve is varied. You can study for vocational awards such as the City & Guilds 6926 Salon Services Certificate (your current course), a National Vocational Qualification (NVQ) or Scottish Vocational Qualification (SVQ) level 1, 2, 3. NVQs and SVQs are the industry standard qualifications.

Specialist qualifications are available from a wide range of awarding bodies, for example aromatherapy qualifications are available from the International Federation of Professional Aromatherapists.

BASIC RIGHTS AND RESPONSIBILITIES OF AN EMPLOYEE

When we go to work we must be aware of what our rights are. There are many regulations and laws designed to ensure that we are not exploited or unfairly treated by our employer. We must also be aware of our responsibilities to our employer. There are laws and regulations that tell us what those responsibilities are.

In this section we will look at some of those rights and regulations. We must remember that these regulations will change and so our rights and responsibilities will change. We must try to keep up to date with these changes. The employer should ensure that you are informed of changes as they may require parts of your job to change.

Our employer has responsibilities to us when we are at work. They include the following:

- The employer must protect us from bullying or harassment.
- They must support us to enable us to carry out our work.
- They must have a procedure to deal with grievances.
- They must provide reasonable, suitable and tolerable working conditions.
- They must pay wages for work done.
- They must provide work for us to earn money (after we are employed).
- They have a duty of care (remember the Health and Safety at Work Act).

As an employee we have duties to our employer; these include the following:

REMEMBER

The Connexions Service will help you find opportunities to advance your career.

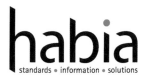

Habia

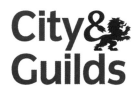

City & Guilds

REMEMBER

Having the right qualifications can open doors to new directions in developing your career.

Make sure that you take those that are necessary for your career plans.

REMEMBER

It is important that we know what we are entitled to when at work and also what our employer is entitled to from us when we are at work.

- We have a duty of trust and confidence, we must show our employer that we are reliable and capable of doing our job.
- We must obey the instructions of our employer as long as they are lawful and reasonable.
- We must work with reasonable care and skill, safely and efficiently.
- We must be loyal and not do the same type of work elsewhere that is not part of this job (without permission).
- We must keep all things about our current job and work confidential, even when we leave and go to work elsewhere.

In Chapter 4, Following Health and Safety Practice, we looked at a number of regulations, such as Personal Protective Equipment at Work Regulations (1992). The main regulations we will look at here are the:

- European Work Time Directive Regulations
- **Disability Discrimination Act**

Some of these will determine how we should conduct ourselves when we are at work.

An important aspect of life today is discrimination. All people have the right not to be unfairly treated or discriminated against for any reason in the course of their employment. This act also applies to other situations. It covers discrimination because of **ethnic origin**, religion, disability, age, full-time and part-time work and more. We, individually, have a responsibility under the act not to discriminate against others.

All employees have a right to join a trade union if they wish to. Trade unions are organisations that provide advice, support and help to employees if they have problems with their employment. Other organisations you could seek advice from would include the Citizens Advice Bureau (CAB), a solicitor and a number of government agencies.

CONFIDENTIALITY

In Chapter 1, Finding out about Customer Service we talked about confidentiality. Our employer will hold information about us. Things like our private address, date of birth, details of our pay and tax payments, other payments, details of any criminal convictions we may have had. Under the requirements of the Data Protection Act this must be kept confidential. It must also be kept up to date and be relevant to why it is recorded. If your information changes, for example if you move, you must give your employer your new address.

Find out more about the Data Protection Act.

THE TERMS AND CONDITIONS OF YOUR EMPLOYMENT

When we get a job we will agree what are called the 'terms and conditions' of the employment, how much pay we will get, what hours we have to work, where we have to work and more. To make sure we agreed all the important

ACTIVITY 009–3

Find out what the word 'discrimination' means.

Make sure your tutor has checked your work. Tick when you have completed this activity.

KEY FACT !

While we all have the right not to be discriminated against, we must remember that we have a duty not to discriminate against others.

ACTIVITY 009–4

Find out about, and write brief notes about, the Data Protection Act.

Make sure your tutor has checked your work. Tick when you have completed this activity.

things about the terms of our employment the employer is required to give us those details in writing. This is called a '**contract of employment**'. It will include details of the following:

- The job you are employed to do e.g. apprenticed hairdresser, beauty therapist.
- It can give details about the range of tasks you will do, but this is not always necessary.
- The name of the employer and the employee.
- The date the employment started.
- The hours and place of work.
- The pay you will receive and how it is calculated.
- Arrangements for sickness pay, pension and holiday entitlement.
- The notice period required if the employment is ended.
- Your job title and brief description of the job.

The 'contract of employment' should be given to you within two months of starting work. You should make sure that you get it, it is an important document that you should keep safe. If you then have a problem it can be used to help resolve the problem quickly.

If your terms and conditions are changed such as your hours of work, your pay, or any of the other things, then your 'contract of employment' should also be changed.

There are a number of other regulations that affect employment. One important set of regulations is the European Work Time Directive. This is part of European legislation and because we are part of the **EU** it affects us. It lays down the maximum number of hours that people should work, particularly young people. Currently no young person under the age of 18 can work more that 40 hours per week. The regulations also ensure employees get paid holiday every year and rest breaks after working a number of hours. Other regulations lay down minimum rates of pay per hour for all employees, whatever work you undertake, young people under 18 have different minimum pay rates. Maternity and paternity leave and sick pay regulations are also covered. **These regulations are changed quite frequently so keeping yourself up to date could be useful.** An employer is required to keep up to date and make sure that all your entitlements are provided.

One thing to remind ourselves of is the nature of the work we do, as we have said before to succeed we have to be flexible. Our clients are our success and so we must make every effort to give them the quality of service they want. As people are involved in our work, things will not always go smoothly, clients will be early, clients will be late, they may come in to the salon at the wrong time and on the wrong day. Others may telephone and need something done in a hurry because of an important event they have to go to. We should be prepared to deal with all of these 'difficulties' even if it means we have to have a short lunch break or work later than we expected. We will be able to take what we have missed some other time.

KEY FACT

We are not always entitled to what we think we are entitled to. Make sure you know what you are entitled to for things like holidays, breaks etc.

REMEMBER

Being flexible about working hours, breaks etc. will enable you to meet your clients' requirements and improve your success.

Key facts for you to remember from this chapter

- To develop a successful career you will need to get qualifications, knowledge and skills, and keep them up to date.

- Know where you can get advice about developing your career.

- Know what opportunities are available to you.

- Being flexible and contributing to the work of the team are essential to your success.

- Have a plan for the development of your career and update it when necessary.

- You should ensure that you get your 'contract of employment' within weeks of starting work.

- Make sure you keep up to date on regulations that affect your working conditions.

- Make sure you know what responsibilities you have to your employer.

GLOSSARY

Aromatherapy A technique of massage using essential oils

Colourist A hairdresser that specialises in hair colouring.

Contract of employment A written statement of the terms and conditions of a person's employment.

Disability Discrimination Act (DDA) The act that makes it illegal to discriminate against other people on a wide variety of grounds.

Electrolysis The permanent removal of unwanted hair.

Ethnic origin A person's race and where they are from.

EU Stands for the European Union, of which the UK is a member.

Health farm A hotel-type complex that specialises in hairdressing, beauty therapy and health fitness including dietary treatments.

Holistic therapists Therapists who specialise in treatments such as aromatherapy, reflexology, reiki (a type of massage), Indian head massage.

Permer A hairdresser who specialises in perming hair.

Reflexology A technique of massaging the feet to improve general health of the whole body.

Training provider An organisation that provides training opportunities for young people, usually through the apprenticeship route.

Trichologist A person who is a specialist in the diagnosis and treatment of hair and scalp disorders.

Questions to test your knowlege of this unit

These are multiple-choice questions. Read the question carefully and then read the four possible answers. When you have decided which of the possible answers is the right one underline either a, b, c, or d in the box under the question.

1 Information about qualifications can be obtained from

   a An awarding body

   b The citizens advice bureau

   c A newspaper

   d A friend

a	b	c	d

2 Where would you find details of the hours you are allowed to work?

   a European Work Time Directive

   b Hours of work regulations

   c Maternity pay regulations

   d Equal pay act

a	b	c	d

3 If you take an apprenticeship in a salon you will be called

   a An assistant

   b A junior

   c An aide

   d A helper

a	b	c	d

4 Which of the following is not normally a recognised salon position

   a Cutter

   b Stylist

   c Beauty therapist

   d Plaiter

a	b	c	d

5 Which of the following is not a reason for discrimination

   a Religion

   b Ethnic origin

   c Disability

   d Colour of hair

a	b	c	d

Questions to test your knowlege of this unit (cont.)

Now try the following short answer questions. These may need a single word to answer or a short sentence or list.

1 Name three places where hairdressing or beauty therapy jobs would be available.

Answer   1. _____

2. _____

3. _____

2 Why should we have a contract of employment?

Answer   _____

_____

3 Why must we try to be flexible about how we work?

Answer   _____

_____

4 Name two ways you could train to be a hairdresser or a beauty therapist.

Answer   1. _____

2. _____

5 Name three specialist jobs you could do after your basic training.

Answer   1. _____

2. _____

3. _____

Helpful hints for the assignment

Introduction to the assignment

This assignment links to all the others in this award, and you should be able to collect information for it while completing the other assignments. It looks at working in the industry, finding out about jobs and careers and about your rights and responsibilities as an employee in a salon.

Your tutor will give you the assignment and guide you on the maximum time you should allow to be sure of completing all of the course assignments.

Organisations providing information about working in the hair and beauty industry

These are going to include: the Internet, magazines like Hairdressers' Journal and even asking hairdressers, beauty therapists and your tutor. When you have some names find out about the organisation, what it does and how it works.

Like you did for your other assignments, make some rough notes about the organisations. You could use some material you have printed from the Internet or leaflets you have collected, so think how you are going to include them in your report. Decide whether you want to use a computer, or write it by hand. You should start with an introduction explaining what you are going to do and what you are going to find out. Then put in your information and pictures. Complete your report with some conclusions; for example, which organisations provide the most information and which awarding body is the most used by the industry.

Jobs in salons and the skills: qualities that salons look for

Don't forget that you will need to find out a lot of detail about one particular job. It might be useful to pick a job that you would like to do in the future.

Make use of the information in this chapter to help you and, once again, some websites could help. Some of the information about jobs and careers could be used again for this task.

You will need to find out things such as; what you would need to do to get the job, what you would have to do when you do the job, and perhaps something about what this particular job could lead to.

As for your other assignments, make rough notes, decide on how you are going to present them and don't forget your introduction and conclusion.

Salon staff structures

You have to produce a report on these structures and how the different jobs relate to each other. You need to write a brief description of what each level of staff does.

There may be some websites that can provide information about staff roles, as could trade magazines. You may also find it helpful to talk to a hairdresser, a beauty therapist or a salon owner. Some of the information in this chapter and from your work on jobs and careers will also be useful for this task.

Again make rough notes, decide on how you are going to present them and don't forget your introduction and conclusion.

Your employment rights and responsibilities as an employee

A lot of the information you need for your outline report (which means brief notes) is in this chapter. You will also find information in the library and some websites. Make sure you cover all of the things listed in the assignment notes. You could also use information from your work on careers, jobs and staff structures, if it is relevant.

Again make rough notes, decide on how you are going to present them and don't forget your introduction and conclusion.

To finish your assignment

When you have most of your information complete, think about the folder you will put it into. Think about the design of the front cover. Another useful thing to do is to get someone to read what you have done to see if it makes sense and provides the information asked for.

Remember you must make a list of where you got your information:

- If it comes from of a book, then give the name of the book, the author, the publisher and the ISBN number (you will find this information on the inside front cover).
- If it is a website then the web address (e.g. www.whatever.com)
- Include a salon name and the owner's name where they provided you with information.
- You don't need to list the names of all the people you asked questions to.

CHECKERBOARD

After you have completed the chapter on Industry and Occupation Awareness rate yourself on the checkerboard. (You must be honest with yourself, don't put a tick in the box if you haven't done the work or don't feel that you have learned what you need to know.)

I am aware of a range of career opportunities open to me ☐	I understand the staffing structures of hair and beauty salons ☐	I am aware of specialist career routes in hairdressing and beauty therapy ☐	I know where I can get information about qualifications ☐
I am aware of the range of qualifications available to me ☐	I understand what the Connexions Service provides ☐	I understand the basic principles of discrimination in the workplace ☐	I know where I can seek advice about employment issues ☐
I know what a 'contract of employment' is and when I should receive one ☐	I know what is contained in a contract of employment ☐	I know about the regulations that affect my employment rights ☐	I understand why I need to be flexible in my approach to working conditions ☐

CHECKER BOARD ✓

ACTIVITY CHECKLIST

Make sure you have completed all the activities linked to this chapter and that you have put any information you need to keep in your portfolio.

Only tick the box and complete the portfolio reference when your tutor has confirmed the activity is complete.

	Complete	Portfolio Reference
Activity 009–1 (p. 153)		
Activity 009–2 (p. 153)		
Activity 009–3 (p. 157)		
Activity 009–4 (p. 157)		

index

Habia series

HAIRDRESSING

Mahogany Hairdressing: Steps to Cutting, Colouring and Finishing Hair *Martin Gannon and Richard Thompson*

Mahogany Hairdressing: Advanced Looks *Richard Thompson and Martin Gannon*

Professional Men's Hairdressing *Guy Kremer and Jacki Wadeson*

The Art of Dressing Long Hair *Guy Kremer and Jacki Wadeson*

Patrick Cameron: Dressing Long Hair *Patrick Cameron and Jacki Wadeson*

Patrick Cameron: Dressing Long Hair Book 2 *Patrick Cameron*

Bridal Hair *Pat Dixon and Jacki Wadeson*

Trevor Sorbie: Visions in Hair *Kris Sorbie and Jacki Wadeson*

The Total Look: The Style Guide for Hair and Make-Up Professionals *Ian Mistlin*

Art of Hair Colouring *David Adams and Jacki Wadeson*

Begin Hairdressing: The Official Guide to Level 1 2e *Martin Green*

Hairdressing – The Foundations: The Official Guide to Level 2 5e *Leo Palladino* (contribution Jane Farr)

Professional Hairdressing: The Official Guide to Level 3 4e *Martin Green, Lesley Kimber and Leo Palladino*

Men's Hairdressing: Traditional and Modern Barbering 2e *Maurice Lister*

African-Caribbean Hairdressing 2e *Sandra Gittens*

Salon Management *Martin Green*

eXtensions: The Official Guide to Hair Extensions *Theresa Bullock*

Trevor Sorbie: The Bridal Hair Book *Trevor Sorbie and Jacki Wadeson*

The Colour Book: The Official Guide to Colour for Levels 2 and 3 *Tracey Lloyd with Christine McMillan-Bodell*

The World of Hair Colour *Dr John Gray*

Hairdressing – The Foundations: Lecturer's Resource Pack, The Official Guide to Level 2 *Jane Farr*

Habia series

BEAUTY THERAPY

Beauty Basics – The Official Guide to Level 1 *Lorraine Nordmann*

Beauty Therapy – The Foundations: The Official Guide to Level 2 3e *Lorraine Nordmann*

Professional Beauty Therapy: The Official Guide to Level 3 2e *Lorraine Nordmann, Lorraine Williamson, Pamela Linforth and Jo Crowder*

Aromatherapy for the Beauty Therapist *Valerie Ann Worwood*

Indian Head Massage 2e *Muriel Burnham-Airey and Adele O'Keefe*

The Official Guide to Body Massage 2e *Adele O'Keefe*

An Holistic Guide to Anatomy and Physiology *Tina Parsons*

The Encyclopedia of Nails 2e *Jacqui Jefford and Anne Swain*

Nail Artistry *Jacqui Jefford, Sue Marsh and Anne Swain*

The Complete Nail Technician 2e *Marian Newman*

The World of Skin Care: A Scientific Companion *Dr John Gray*

Safety in the Salon *Elaine Almond*

An Holistic Guide to Reflexology *Tina Parsons*

Nutrition: A Practical Approach *Suzanne Le Quesne*

An Holistic Guide to Massage *Tina Parsons*

The Spa Book: The Official Guide to Spa Therapy *Jane Crebbin-Bailey, Dr John Harcup and John Harrington*

The Art of Nails: A Comprehensive Style Guide to Nail Treatments and Nail Art *Jacqui Jefford*

The Complete Guide to Make-up *Suzanne LeQuesne*

The Essential Guide to Holistic and Complementary Therapy *Helen Beckmann and Suzanne LeQuesne*

Hands On Sports Therapy *Kevin Ward*

Manicure, Pedicure and Advanced Nail Techniques *Elaine Almond*

Complete Make-up Artist: Working in Film, Fashion, Television and Theatre 2e *Penny Delamar*